MENOPAUSE

First published in September 2019
Reprinted 2019 (twice), 2020 (twice) and 2021 (four times)

British Library Cataloguing in Publication Data
A catalogue record for this book is available
from the British Library.

ISBN 978 1 78521 642 8

Library of Congress catalog card no. 2019934662

Published by J H Haynes & Co. Ltd.,
Sparkford, Yeovil, Somerset BA22 7JJ, UK
Tel: 01963 440635
Int. tel: +44 1963 440635
Website: www.haynes.com

Haynes North America Inc.,
859 Lawrence Drive, Newbury Park,
California 91320, USA

Page design and layout: Richard Parsons

Printed and bound in Malaysia

Images
Laura May Photography - page 2 middle, 6, 47, 70, 87, back cover bottom.
Simon Russell – pages 32, 34, 42 and 78
All other images from Shutterstock

MENOPAUSE

ALL YOU NEED TO KNOW IN ONE CONCISE MANUAL

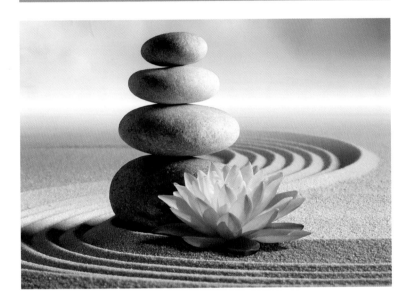

Dr Louise Newson

Contents

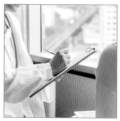
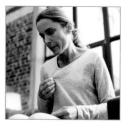
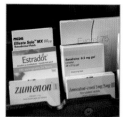

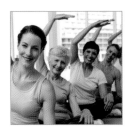
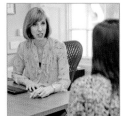
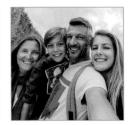

Introduction

Menopause is a completely normal, natural event that every woman – including you (unless you are a man reading this!) – will go through, yet it remains a subject shrouded in secrecy.

As a menopause specialist, I run a dedicated menopause and wellbeing centre where we help thousands of women each year whose lives are being blighted by symptoms such as hot flushes, mood changes, anxiety, brain fog and vaginal dryness. The transformation within a few months of accessing the right support and treatment is often nothing short of remarkable.

My working life revolves around the menopause: running my clinic, delivering menopause training to general practitioners (GPs) and nurses, updating the My Menopause Doctor website (www.menopausedoctor.co.uk) and helping the media to give the right information about the menopause to women. But as a doctor, and as a woman, I'm often dismayed at the lack of accurate information about the menopause online, in the media and even in some GP consulting rooms.

First, there's confusion over symptoms, with so many women blaming the early warning signs on the stresses and strains of everyday life. Then there's confusion over the safety of treatments. Hormone replacement therapy (HRT) remains the most effective treatment for troublesome symptoms, yet women are often wary of taking it. This means that in some parts of the UK only one in ten women who would benefit from taking HRT actually take it.[1]

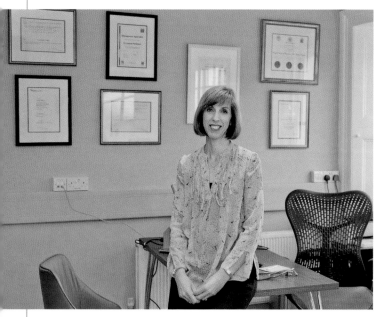

← At my dedicated menopause and wellbeing centre we help thousands of women to experience the best possible menopause.

There are many excellent healthcare professionals out there giving superb care for menopausal women, yet a lack of menopause training means that there are still those who are not up to speed on the latest evidence and treatment guidelines. I was a GP for 18 years and I know that practices are under immense pressure. However, too many women are being given outdated advice or are being refused treatment that could really make a difference, as the findings of my survey of almost 3,000 women show (see box).

This has to change. I'm passionate that every woman, including you, has access to clear information so you can make an informed choice about the right treatment and support to allow you to have the best possible menopause. In this manual I'll cover:

◆ Symptoms to look out for and long-term health implications.
◆ Myth-busting HRT.
◆ Alternative treatments if HRT isn't for you.
◆ How to get the best out of your medical appointment.
◆ Holistic therapies and the importance of a balanced diet and exercise.

Good menopause care is not just about managing the physical symptoms. I've lost count of the number of women who have sat in my consulting room and tearfully told me how their symptoms have affected their relationships and love lives, and how they can't bring themselves to talk about it. I've sympathised with partners and family members who tell me they feel powerless and have no idea how to help the women they love.

Too many women think they must

Women's menopause care

I surveyed almost 2,920 women about their experiences of menopause care. The majority of respondents had visited their usual GP, and findings included:

◆ 66% of women said they were offered antidepressants instead of HRT.
◆ 20% said they had been referred to a hospital for appointments and/or investigations that are likely to be related to their perimenopause/menopause, such as migraine clinics, scans or heart tests.
◆ Just 28% said a healthcare professional had discussed lifestyle choices in relation to their perimenopause or menopause.
◆ The overall rating for receiving evidence-based, non-biased care was 2.5 out of 5.

simply soldier on through troublesome symptoms. This 'put up with it' mentality not only risks ruining relationships, but careers too, with one in ten women admitting they have considered quitting their job because of their symptoms.[2]

It doesn't have to be like this. That's why this manual is packed with advice and coping strategies to safeguard your relationships at home and in the workplace.

Throughout this manual will be advice for those around you: for your partners, children, employers and co-workers. Together we can bring the menopause issue out in the open so all women can access the right support and make the 'change' a positive one.

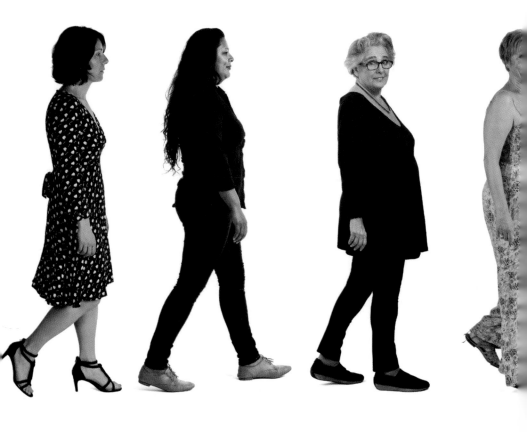

Chapter 1
Menopause 101

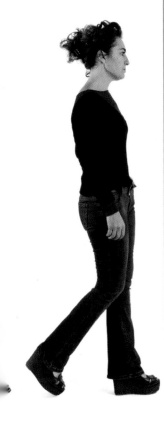

The mere mention of the word 'menopause' often causes confusion. Society's reluctance to discuss the menopause openly, misinformation in the media and a lack of credible information online mean that many of us just don't know what to expect. By far the best way you can prepare for your menopause is by familiarising yourself with the facts. This chapter covers the essentials, including:

◆ Why your menopause happens.
◆ When and how it happens.
◆ How you can get a diagnosis from your doctor or healthcare professional with an interest in menopause.
◆ How long your menopause may last for.

Arming yourself with this knowledge will help you to recognise the signs and symptoms of your menopause and, crucially, will help you to feel empowered to ask for help in coping with the symptoms should you need to.

What is the menopause?

How will I know it is happening? Why do I feel so shattered all the time? Will I ever feel like 'me' again? These may be just some of the questions you might have right now.

The age you will go through your menopause and your symptoms depends on a host of factors including genetics, any underlying conditions, surgery or treatments. I'm afraid there is no crystal ball to predict exactly when your menopause will happen for you and which symptoms you will experience.

Sure, everyone knows that you can get hot flushes, but do you know why they happen, and how you can get help? It is vital you know about the potential symptoms, so you can recognise what your own body is telling you when the time comes.

What is your menopause?

Put simply, your menopause is when you stop having periods and are no longer able to get pregnant naturally. However, the actual definition of being menopausal is when you have not had a period for one year.

Why does it happen: thank your hormones

Women have two ovaries – grape-sized glands that lie either side of your uterus. The ovaries have two main functions. They release an egg each month during the menstrual cycle for possible fertilisation, a process known as ovulation. The ovaries also produce hormones, which are chemical messengers that travel through our bloodstream to our tissues and organs affecting processes such as growth and development, sexual function, reproduction and mood. The ovaries produce three key types of hormones:

- **Estrogen:** an umbrella term for three female sex hormones that have a number of functions in every part of our body.

- **Progesterone:** this hormone helps to maintain the menstrual cycle and is an important hormone during pregnancy.

- **Testosterone:** although it is commonly seen as a 'male' hormone, women also produce testosterone. Testosterone is also produced in the adrenal glands.

What happens to my hormones during menopause?

Your menopause occurs when your ovaries stop producing eggs and, as a result, the levels of estrogen, progesterone and testosterone fall.

Did you know?

The word menopause actually means your last menstrual period – 'meno' refers to your menstrual cycle, and 'pause' literally means stop.

How hormones affect your body

Brain

Estrogen
Helps to regulate mood and body temperature, maintains memory and cognition

Testosterone
Regulates sex drive. Can improve mood, concentration, memory and sense of wellbeing

Reproductive system

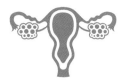

Estrogen
Maintains menstrual cycle and lubricates the vagina

Progesterone
Maintains the menstrual cycle, prepares the uterus (womb) for and supports the body during pregnancy

Heart

Estrogen
Protects the arteries

Breasts

Estrogen
Stimulates breast growth during puberty

Bones, muscles and joints

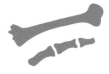

Estrogen
Helps stimulate bone growth, maintains strength, lubricates the joints

Testosterone
Helps to improve bone growth, strength and muscle mass

Perimenopause

During a natural menopause our ovaries won't suddenly stop working, rather they will slow down over time. The transition period right before your menopause begins is called the perimenopause. For many women this starts at around 45 years of age,[3] and it is the time where you still have periods, but they may be more irregular or lighter than you are used to. You may also experience menopausal symptoms (such as hot flushes and mood swings) during this time.

How can I be suffering symptoms without actually being in the menopause?

Estrogen and progesterone work together to regulate your menstrual cycle and also the production of eggs. During the perimenopause, the levels of these hormones fluctuate greatly and it is often the imbalance of these hormones which

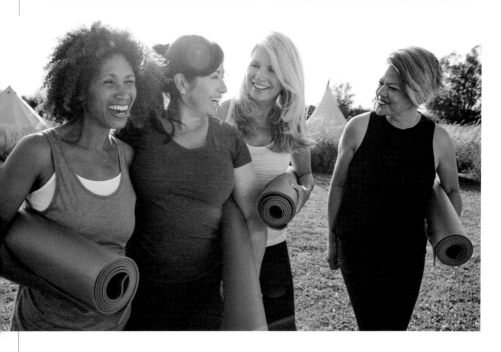

My menopause story

Believe me, I know from personal experience about the importance of listening to your body. Despite my background as a GP and a menopause specialist, I am embarrassed to admit that I failed to recognise my own menopausal symptoms; it was my then-11-year-old daughter who actually made the diagnosis for me.

I had been experiencing horrendous night sweats most nights for a few months. Waking up in the early hours of the morning covered in a layer of sweat was awful. Some nights I would wake up worried that I had wet the bed as the sheets around me were wringing. Changing my pyjamas and the bed sheets once or twice a night was doing nothing for my husband's mood and energy levels, nor our relationship.

I also experienced extreme fatigue similar to the tiredness I felt when pregnant. I was also finding it impossible to concentrate on even the simplest of tasks. I blamed the extra demands of work and life in general so hadn't really thought much about there being another cause for these symptoms.

My joints had become stiff and my muscles were sore so I had reduced the frequency of exercise, including yoga, which I love. I have always had migraines, but these were coming closer together and far more painful and debilitating. I was also more anxious than I had ever been and I generally felt flat and low in my mood. Life was less pleasurable in general for me.

Then, a few months later, I was cooking in the kitchen and experienced my first hot flush; it was unbearable! One of my daughters asked me what was wrong as I looked so hot and sweaty. Then she asked me why I had been so short-tempered and irritable with her and all the family recently. She even asked if I was due my period as her friends were quite often stroppy before their periods.

It was only then that the penny dropped and I realised I hadn't actually had a period for several months. I was 45 years old and although perimenopausal symptoms can often occur in women from this age, I just wasn't expecting them to happen to me. I felt so stupid but this gave me a real insight as to how many women can easily dismiss their symptoms as being due to the general stresses and strains of life.

leads to symptoms of the menopause, such as hot flushes, night sweats, joint and muscle pain, vaginal dryness, mood changes and a lack of interest in sex. This is because estrogen protects a number of different systems in your body; your brain, skin, bones, heart and vagina – low levels can affect all these parts of your body.

How long will be I be perimenopausal for?

Every woman is different. I have treated women who have experienced symptoms for a couple of months, others have been plagued for several years or even decades before their periods finally stop. Once you have not had a period for 12 consecutive months, then you are in the menopause.

Keep a note in your diary or phone each month that you don't have a period. It can be helpful to refer to these notes when you see your doctor or healthcare professional with an interest in menopause.

How old will I be when I reach the menopause?

The average age of the menopause for UK women is 51,[3] but genetics, underlying medical conditions and treatment for cancer can mean that you go through it at an earlier age.

If the menopause occurs when you are under 45 years of age then it is called an early menopause. If you are under 40 it is known as a premature menopause, or premature ovarian insufficiency (POI).

Menopausal symptoms under 40?

POI affects about one in a hundred women under 40 in the UK.[4] It occurs when your ovaries no longer produce normal amounts of estrogen and therefore may not produce eggs. This means that your periods will become irregular or stop altogether, and you may experience symptoms of the menopause.

Many women have POI without actually realising it, so if you are under 40 and have irregular periods (or if they have even

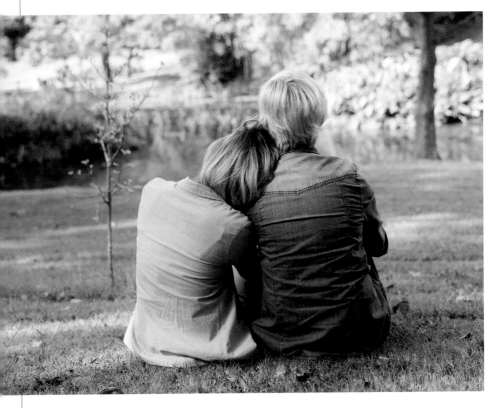

stopped completely) you should be talking to your doctor about having tests. No woman is too young to be menopausal.

Unlike the normal menopause when the ovaries stop working completely, in POI ovarian function can be intermittent, occasionally resulting in a period, ovulation or even pregnancy. This intermittent return of ovarian function means that 5–10% of women with POI are able to conceive.[4]

My mum went through an early menopause: does that mean I will too?

Many women I see in my clinic have been told by their previous doctor that they are 'too young' to be menopausal – clearly this is not true. Although POI and early menopause are not hereditary, many women who have an early menopause find that other family female members have also had an early menopause. So it is always worth asking your mother, grandmother, aunts, sisters and cousins if they had an early menopause so you can prepare yourself for the possibility.

Surgical menopause: what you need to know

If you undergo a hysterectomy (an operation to remove your uterus) you may also have your ovaries removed at the same time. If this happens then you will immediately be put into the menopause, an event known as a surgical menopause, regardless of age.

Even if one or both of your ovaries are left intact following a hysterectomy, there is a chance that you will experience the menopause within five years of having the operation.[5] Although your ovaries will still make some estrogen after your hysterectomy, commonly, your level

Other menopause triggers

Although there is no obvious underlying cause for an early menopause or POI to occur in most women, certain conditions can bring about an early menopause, including:

◆ An underlying medical condition, such as Addison's disease or Down's syndrome.

◆ An autoimmune disease, such as type 1 diabetes.

◆ Infection, such as mumps (although this is very uncommon).

◆ Cancer treatment such as radiotherapy to your pelvic area, or certain types of chemotherapy that negatively affect ovarian function.

of estrogen will fall at an earlier age than average.

Medical or surgical treatment for endometriosis or premenstrual syndrome may also trigger an early menopause.

What about my fertility?

The 2015 National Institute for Health and Care Excellence (or NICE) menopause guidelines recommend that if you are due to have treatment that is likely to cause the menopause, then your doctor should explain to you what you should expect and how it will affect your fertility. You should also be offered support and information about how to manage your menopause if your treatment is going to lead to the menopause occurring.[6]

How is my menopause diagnosed?

If menopausal symptoms are affecting your day-to-day life you should see your doctor or a healthcare professional with an interest in the menopause. They should be able to tell if you are in perimenopause or menopause based on your age, symptoms and how often you have periods, so you are unlikely to need tests.

Hormone blood tests vary tremendously and are a very unreliable way of testing for the menopause. The NICE menopause guidelines are very clear that women do not need to have a hormone blood test to diagnose their menopause when they have symptoms and are over 45 years of age.[7]

Sometimes health professionals carry out blood tests to ensure that there is no other underlying cause for your symptoms (for example an underactive thyroid) or to assess actual estrogen or testosterone blood levels. This is not the same as having a blood test to diagnose the perimenopause or menopause, which is not necessary. However, blood tests may be useful in some circumstances:

◆ If you are younger than 45 years of age and are experiencing menopausal symptoms. The most common test is a blood test measuring a level of a hormone called follicle-stimulating hormone (FSH), which is often found in higher levels during the menopause. This blood test is often repeated after four to six weeks.

⇩ Hormone blood tests are an unreliable way to test for the the menopause.

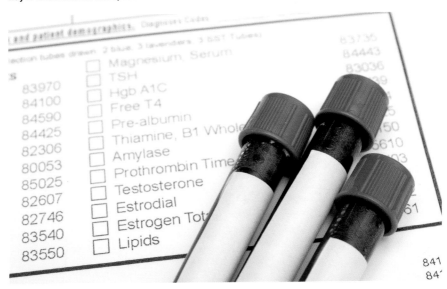

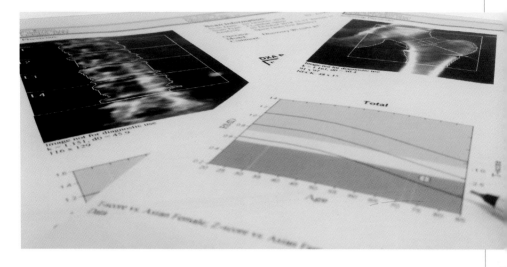

- If you are under 40 years you may be advised to have additional blood tests to try to determine if there is an underlying cause for your early menopause.
- Falling levels of estrogen can affect your bones, so younger women may also be recommended to have a bone density test (called a DEXA scan, or dual-energy X-ray absorptiometry) to determine the strength of your bones. DEXA scans can be hard to access on the NHS, but in an ideal world I strongly feel that every woman should have a DEXA scan to assess her underlying bone mineral density, as osteoporosis is so common in menopausal women and is often not diagnosed until a fracture occurs.

↑ Falling estrogen can affect your bones, so a bone density test may be recommended for some women.

general. So, for example, some women find that hot flushes and night sweats (known as vasomotor symptoms) improve with time, and then they develop other symptoms such as poor sleep and worsening anxiety.

Even if you have not experienced troublesome symptoms during your menopause, your body will still have to contend with the effects of low hormone levels, which can have a detrimental impact on your future health, including increased risk of osteoporosis and cardiovascular disease.

How long will my menopause last?

Most women can expect to experience symptoms for about four years after their last period, but one in ten women can experience them for up to 12 years.[8] Symptoms often change with time, so it can sometimes be difficult to know which symptoms are due to changing hormone levels and which are related to life in

What does postmenopausal mean?

The postmenopause is the time in your life after your actual menopause, so any time from a year after your last period. On average, women spend one-third of their life postmenopausal.[9] This is very different to Victorian times, when the average age for a woman's menopause was 57 years and her average age at death was 59 years.

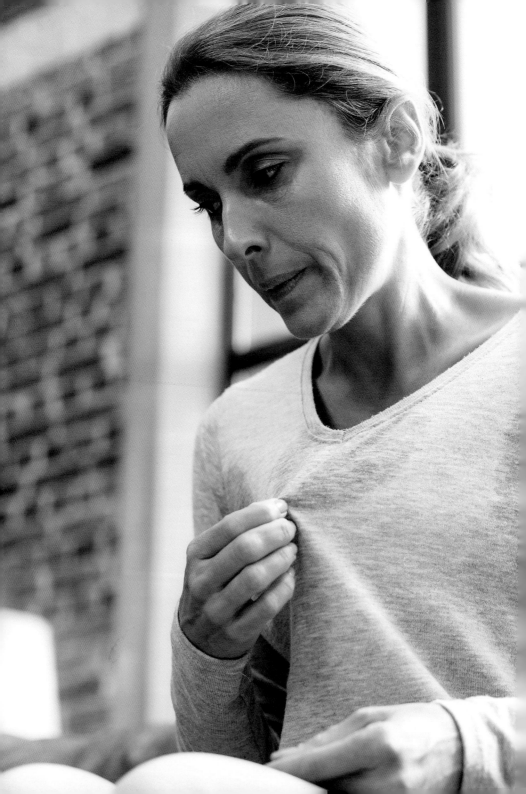

Chapter 2
Menopause symptoms

Hot flushes. Night sweats. Weight gain. Most of us know the classic symptoms we can expect during our perimenopause and menopause. But this hormonal rollercoaster can throw up some surprising symptoms, including aching joints, a burning mouth, heart palpitations, tingling skin – even the acne you thought you'd left behind in your teenage years.

This chapter covers a comprehensive list of symptoms that can occur during your perimenopause and menopause, and why they happen. Thankfully, you won't usually experience every single one, but some symptoms can trigger others – as in the case of night sweats and poor sleep, for example.

You may well be affected by some of the symptoms listed here, but it is really important to be aware of the full range of symptoms, so take some time to read through them all before moving on to what treatments can bring relief in the following chapters.

Hormonal rollercoaster

Cells throughout our body thrive on estrogen. And when levels of estrogen (and progesterone and testosterone) fluctuate and fall during the perimenopause and menopause, this can trigger changes throughout our entire system.

As we know, every woman's menopause experience is different. Some women experience more physical symptoms, others suffer more with psychological symptoms, whereas others experience both. As your hormone levels change, it can be common for symptoms to come and go. So what sort of symptoms can be put down to your menopause?

Changes to your periods

Chances are that the first real sign of your perimenopause/menopause will be changes to your periods. Fluctuating hormone levels may cause your periods to become lighter or even heavier than you are used to. You may find they become less frequent, before tailing off and eventually stopping altogether.

Hot flushes

Hot flushes are the most common and instantly recognisable symptom, affecting three in four women. A hot flush is often a feeling of intense heat that comes on suddenly and spreads throughout your face, neck, chest and body.

Women I have treated and spoken to describe it as an abnormal sensation that occurs, often over the top of their body or head, which can last for seconds or minutes. Many women tell me that they feel cold before the actual flush occurs. Some women also sweat but some just flush. During a hot flush, you may experience:

- flushing of your face
- sweating
- dizziness/feeling light-headed
- heart palpitations.

Hot flushes can last anything from a matter of seconds or up to an hour. Some women may have hot flushes a few times a month, while others endure several a day. Most women can expect to experience hot flushes for about four years, while some may have to cope with them for decades.[11] I've even seen women in their 70s with these symptoms.

Much debate surrounds the exact of cause of hot flushes, but one theory is that falling estrogen levels impact on another hormone called noradrenaline (also called norepinephrine), which helps to regulate body temperature. Low noradrenaline levels can cause your body core temperature to rise, resulting in a hot flush.[12] Triggers for hot flushes can include spicy foods, hot drinks, caffeine and alcohol.

Night sweats

Like hot flushes, night sweats are also very common. Many women find that they wake up several times a night and are drenched in sweat and may need to change their pyjamas or bedding. Not only is it a horrible symptom for you to endure, but it can also be disruptive to your partner's sleep too.

Symptoms of menopause

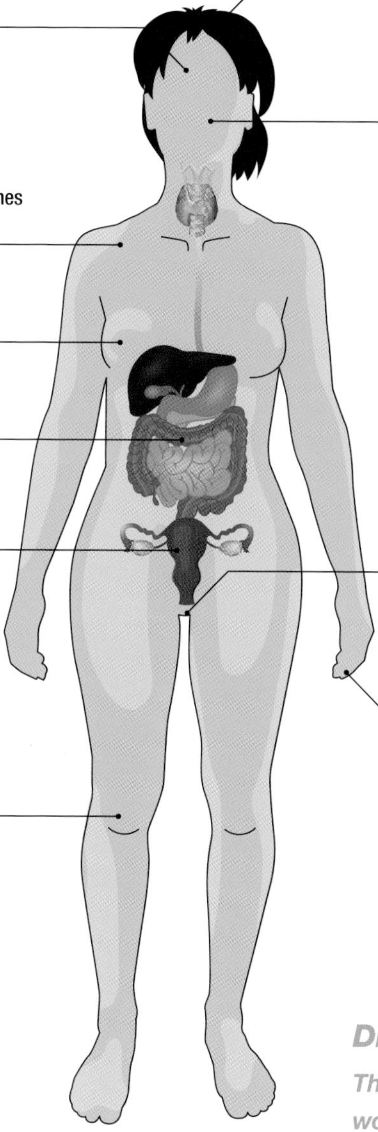

- Brain fog
- Mood changes
- Memory problems
- Low motivation
- Poor concentration
- Migraines and headaches

- Hot flushes
- Night sweats

- Breast pain

- Digestive problems
- Weight gain

- Loss of libido
- Vaginal dryness
- Menstrual periods occur less often and eventually stop

- Joint pain
- Osteoporosis
- Muscle stiffness

- Hair changes (thinning and dryness)

- Dry skin
- Itchiness
- Acne
- Wrinkles
- Altered sense of smell
- Dry eyes
- Facial hair
- Burning mouth
- Dry mouth

- Frequent urination
- Urinary pain
- Incontinence

- Brittle nails

Did you know?

Three in four women suffer from hot flushes.[10]

Mood changes

Your menopause often throws up so many physical symptoms, but for the majority of women I see it is the onset of less spoken about psychological symptoms that are the hardest to cope with. Mood changes are extremely common during your perimenopause and menopause. You may feel quick to anger one minute, tearful the next. These feelings can be distressing, confusing and have a huge effect on your self-confidence and relationships at home and work.

Estrogen helps to regulate serotonin, a neurotransmitter (a messenger chemical) that carries signals between nerve cells in the brain. It is known as the 'feel-good chemical' thanks to its positive effects on mood, emotion, energy and sleep, so falling levels of estrogen can directly impact on your mood. Mood changes you may experience include:

- anger or aggression
- frustration
- irritability
- low self-esteem
- panic
- poor motivation/feeling disinterested
- tearfulness.

Many women tell me that they feel joyless, low and frankly fed up, with one summing up her mood as feeling 'as flat as a pancake'. If you have had postnatal depression in the past, or a history of premenstrual syndrome, then it is more likely that you will experience mood change symptoms. This is because your body is more sensitive to changing levels of hormones.

Menopausal mood changes should not be confused with depression. Yet, frustratingly, my survey showed that 66% of the 3,000 women who took part have been offered antidepressants by their doctors.[13] This is despite there being no evidence that they help to improve the low mood associated with the perimenopause and menopause.

Tiredness and insomnia

With fluctuating estrogen levels leading to hot flushes, night sweats and urinary problems to name but a few, it is no wonder that many women find it impossible to get a good night's sleep. Anxiety, stress and depression can also lead to poor sleep and early morning waking.

Progesterone can be beneficial for sleep. This hormone increases the production of GABA (or gamma-aminobutyric acid), another chemical in our brain that works to help sleep.

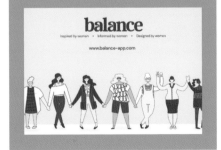

Menopause-proof your bedroom

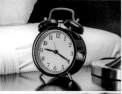

Keep bedtime consistent
Going to sleep and waking up at the same time every day is crucial for setting your body's internal clock (known as your circadian rhythm), according to the US-based National Sleep Foundation (www.sleep.org/articles/design-perfect-bedtime-routine).

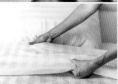

Ditch the heavy duvet
Switch to sheets that can easily be thrown off or a lighter duvet to avoid overheating. And if your partner prefers to be toasty, you could compromise with a split-tog duvet, with two different tog (warmth) ratings on either side.

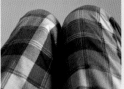

Lose the synthetic nightwear
Invest in some nightwear made from natural fabrics like cotton and bamboo, which keep skin cool by wicking sweat from the body. And keep a spare pair handy in case you need to change.

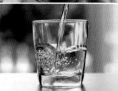

Say no to a cup of cocoa
Hot drinks before bed can cause sweating as the body tries to cool you down. Try water instead. Likewise, avoid stimulants like caffeine or nicotine before bedtime.

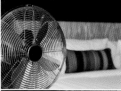

Cool it
A bedside fan is a quick way to get some cooling relief from night sweats.

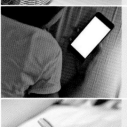

Ban screen time before bed
Devices like smartphones and tablets emit short-wavelength blue light, which can disrupt the sleep hormone melatonin. Getting as much daylight as possible during waking hours also helps to regulate your circadian rhythm.

Mind racing? Write a to do list
Taking five minutes before bedtime to jot down any uncompleted tasks can help induce sleepiness by allowing you to offload your thoughts and worries, according to a study by sleep scientists at Baylor University, Texas.[14]

Progesterone can promote relaxation and help improve mood. Lower levels of progesterone occur during the perimenopause and menopause and this can lead to symptoms such as anxiety, restlessness and trouble sleeping, including a tendency to wake up frequently.

Low testosterone levels can also have a negative effect on sleep duration and quality in women, and melatonin, the hormone which helps to regulate sleep, can be affected by changing estrogen and progesterone levels.

Brain fog and poor concentration

One woman recently described it to me as feeling like a 'blank sheet of paper – my memory and concentration have gone and I am a different person to who I used to be.' Her doctor had even arranged a brain scan to get to the bottom of her symptoms. We have hormone receptors in our brains, so when hormone levels fall, our memory and cognition can be affected.

Worsening migraines

If you have suffered from migraines in the past, you might find fluctuating estrogen levels can cause your migraines to become more severe or closer together. According to the Migraine Trust, the few studies that have been conducted into the subject found that the menopause makes migraine worse for up to 45% of women.[15]

Joint pains

You may notice that your joints can feel stiff and aching; this happens because

⬇ **Low estrogen levels can lead to joint pains and stiffness.**

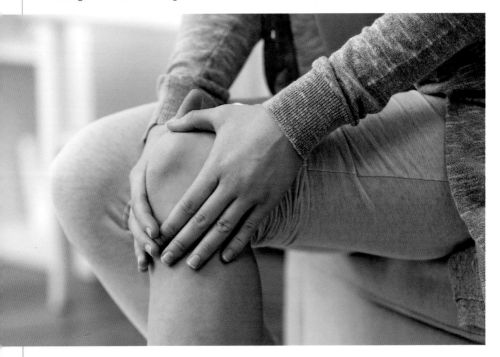

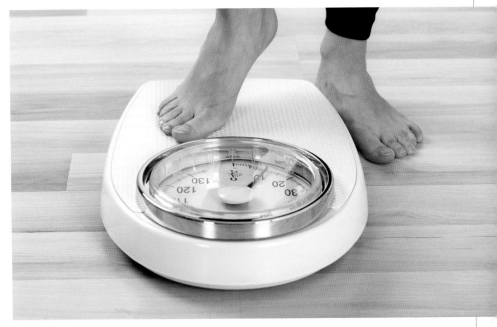

of falling estrogen. That's because the estrogen is hugely important in providing lubrication in your joints. It helps to reduce inflammation and helps keep your bones strong.

Weight gain

Falling estrogen levels can alter the way we store fat and can change our body shape, with greater fat distribution around our middle.[16] Storing fat around the abdomen increases the risk of heart disease, diabetes and cancer.[17] Add menopause-related aching joints, low mood and self-esteem and tiredness to the mix, and it can be easy to skip exercise and reach for sugary foods for a treat or energy boost.

The ageing process also has an effect on our weight. From the age of 40, our muscles lose strength and mass (a process known as sarcopenia). Our metabolism slows, meaning we are more likely to gain fat. Research has shown that our weight can have a bearing on the severity of menopausal symptoms. A study of 749 Brazilian women aged 45–60 revealed that obese women suffered more severe consequences of hot flushes, joint and muscular pain and more intense urinary symptoms.[18]

Reduced sex drive

Changes in our estrogen and testosterone can lead to levels of reduced libido (sex drive), poor arousal and impaired orgasms. Fluctuating hormone levels, coupled with the vaginal dryness and painful sex that can occur, mean that it is no surprise that sex might be the last thing on your mind. If this sounds familiar, then you aren't alone. Around half of the women I see in my menopause clinic tell me that they have not had sex with their partner for at least a year. Many say they still love their partner, they just aren't interested in sex.

Urinary and bladder problems

Many women find that their perimenopause and menopause can lead to embarrassing symptoms including leaking when coughing or sneezing, an urge to go to the toilet more often, constipation and wind due to a weakening pelvic floor. Estrogen plays a key role in maintaining our pelvic floor, a hammock-like layer of muscles stretching from the pubic bone to the bottom of the spine. The pelvic floor muscles help to keep our bowel, bladder and uterus in place and controls the passing of urine, gas and bowel movements. A strong pelvic floor also increases sensitivity and satisfaction during sex.

Aside from the menopause, other factors that can weaken your pelvic floor over time include the effects of pregnancy and childbirth, constipation and being overweight.

Bladder control issues and infections

Lack of estrogen can thin the lining of your bladder and urethra (the tube which carries urine out of your body). These changes to your urinary tract can lead to:

◆ stress incontinence: leaking when the bladder is put under pressure from coughing, sneezing, sudden movements or lifting something heavy
◆ urge incontinence: a sudden, urgent urge to urinate
◆ nocturia: excessive urinating at night.[19]

The urinary tract

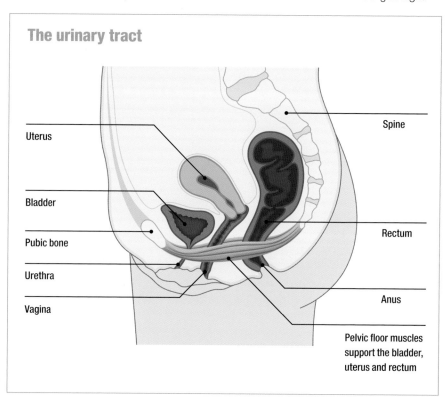

Uterus

Bladder

Pubic bone

Urethra

Vagina

Spine

Rectum

Anus

Pelvic floor muscles support the bladder, uterus and rectum

How to do pelvic floor exercises

Just like any damaged muscle, the pelvic floor muscles need to be exercised to improve strength. These daily lift and squeeze exercises, also known as Kegels, can help restore some of the lost strength.

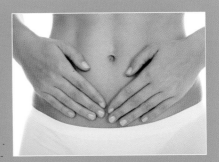

1 Sit or stand with your knees slightly apart.

2 Squeeze the muscles around your bottom as though you are trying to stop yourself passing wind. Then, tighten and lift around your vagina as though you are stopping yourself from peeing.

3 Hold this position for up to 10 seconds, ensuring your buttocks, legs and stomach remain relaxed throughout.

4 Slowly release. Repeat 10 times, resting for 5 seconds between each exercise. Repeat 3 times a day.

You could set an alarm on your phone to remind you to do your exercises, or download the Squeezy app (squeezyapp.com), which is designed by NHS chartered physiotherapists and takes you through the exercises. Always make sure that your bladder is empty before starting the exercises.

When will I see improvements?

Persevere – you should expect to see improvements within a few months. It is important to do these exercises every single day. If you are really struggling, see a health professional, who may be able to refer you to a physiotherapist or a continence service.

You can also be more prone to urinary tract infection (UTI). Symptoms of a UTI include:

◆ needing to urinate suddenly or more often
◆ a burning sensation when urinating
◆ smelly or cloudy urine
◆ tummy pain.

How can I combat these bladder issues?

You should always see a health professional if you think you have an infection or are having recurrent infections. You might need to have a sample of your urine tested for infections or a bladder scan if you have recurrent infections. Cut back on caffeine, but keep drinking water. Caffeine can irritate the bladder further, but don't be tempted to reduce your water intake if you are having accidents. Not drinking enough can make your urine more concentrated, which can irritate the bladder and lead to UTIs.

Squeeze and lift if you feel like you are going to sneeze or cough and when you have to lift something heavy. Avoid exercises that put pressure on the pelvic floor and give high-impact exercises such as aerobics or jogging a miss until your pelvic floor strength improves.

Breast changes

Falling estrogen levels can make the breast tissue dehydrated and less elastic, so you may notice that your breasts lose their rounded shape and start to sag. Lumps in your breasts are also common during the menopause.[20] They are usually harmless, but do see a health professional if you have any concerns.

Heart palpitations

Your menopause can cause palpitations – a feeling that your heart is beating faster – due to changing hormone levels. This can sometimes happen during hot flushes. Palpitations are usually harmless, especially if they disappear when you exercise. If they are frequent or are associated with other symptoms such as shortness of breath then you should see your doctor.

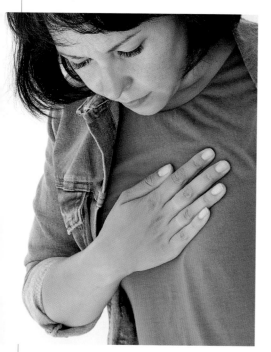

Skin, hair and nail changes

Dry, saggy or wrinkled skin

Estrogen works to build collagen, a connective protein that gives your skin strength and structure. Estrogen is also key in maintaining a blood supply to the upper layer of your skin (known as the epidermis) and keeping it well hydrated and elastic. As estrogen levels fall, you may notice your skin becoming less plump and an increase in fine lines and wrinkles. According to the American Academy of Dermatology, studies show that women's skin loses about 30% of its collagen during the first five years of the menopause.[21]

Itchy skin

Falling estrogen can also result in itchy skin, which can occur day and night and can be really troublesome. Some women notice abnormal sensations to their skin, such as numbness, tingling, prickling or a crawling sensation (called formication).

Acne

You may have thought that you had left spotty skin behind during your teenage years, but some women find they have acne for the first time in decades. Testosterone changes trigger overproduction of a natural oil called sebum. Sebum and dead skin block your hair follicles, resulting in greasy skin and breakouts.

Hair changes

Estrogen is important for hair growth and reducing levels can alter texture of hair, leaving it finer, drier and more brittle. As estrogen falls, androgens (a collective term for male hormones such as testosterone) become more prominent. This can lead to

Will my skin be more sensitive in the sun?

In a word, yes. As estrogen levels fall during your perimenopause and menopause, the number of cells that produce melanin, a pigment which gives our skin colour and protects it from the sun, also falls. This means that menopausal skin can appear lighter and it is more prone to sun damage, so wearing a sunscreen with a high sun protection factor is more important than ever.

If you have been a sun worshipper in the past, you might now start seeing the effects. Estrogen helps to regulate melanin production, but without as much estrogen to keep it in check during your menopause, melanin production increases. This can result in brown age spots appearing in areas of skin that have been exposed to the sun's harmful ultraviolet rays, such as your face, hands, neck, arms and chest. These spots are harmless and should not cause any pain, but if you experience any skin changes that concern you, then please do see a health professional.

the unwanted side effects of excess facial hair around the lip and chin area. Androgens can also shrink our hair follicles, resulting in finer hair that gives less coverage, causing thinning hair on the scalp. You might notice your parting becoming wider. An estimated 40% of women will experience hair loss during and after their menopause, but hair loss can also occur during your perimenopause.[22]

Brittle hair and nails

Estrogen aids the production of keratin, a protein that helps keep our hair, skin and nails strong. You may find that your hair is drier and more prone to breakage.

Altered senses

Smell

Estrogen can affect the pathways in our brains that control sense of smell. Some women initially have a heightened sense of smell others find their sense of smell reduces.

Sight

Dry, itchy, gritty or blurry eyes? It might be dry-eye syndrome. Studies have shown that dry-eye syndrome is more common in women, with menopausal and postmenopausal women most affected.[23] Hormonal changes can mean that you produce fewer tears, which help to keep your eyes lubricated and comfortable.

Taste

A more unusual symptom during your perimenopause or menopause is burning-mouth syndrome, a hot sensation affecting your tongue, lips, gums or inside your cheek. According to the Oral Health Foundation, the exact cause is unknown, but it is thought that hormone changes can trigger it, and it is more common in menopausal and postmenopausal women.[24]

Declining estrogen can reduce moisture in the mucus membranes in the mouth, leading to a dry mouth.

Long-term conditions that can arise from the menopause

Vaginal dryness

Estrogen keeps your vagina healthy by acting as a natural lubricant. It also stimulates the cells in the lining of your vagina to produce glycogen, a compound that encourages the presence of 'good' bacteria to protect your vagina from infections. Low estrogen can thin the tissues lining the vagina, which is known as vaginal atrophy or atrophic vaginitis. This condition can lead to symptoms of dryness, itching and inflammation, and infections such as thrush. You may also find sex painful, as your vagina shrinks a little and expands less easily during sex.

I find that while many women are very open about their struggles with hot flushes, many are reluctant to talk about vaginal dryness. One woman admitted to me that she had not been able to wear trousers for four years because her vaginal dryness made wearing them too painful. The severity of symptoms varies from woman to woman, but vaginal dryness is one symptom that can remain after the menopause. Symptoms often worsen with time as, once the tissues are thin, they don't repair and regenerate without the estrogen to replace them. In Chapter 6, we cover how different treatments like moisturisers and lubricants can help with vaginal dryness.

Osteoporosis

Osteoporosis is a condition that weakens our bones, making them more likely to break – even from a simple fall. Bone is a living tissue that regenerates throughout our lives. Our bodies are constantly laying down new bone and removing old bone to keep our bones strong and healthy. Up to about 30 years of age, we normally build more bone than we lose, but after then our bone tissue naturally starts to decrease.

Why am at I at increased risk of osteoporosis?

During your menopause, bone breakdown occurs more rapidly than bone build-up. About 10% of a woman's bone mass is lost in the first five years of the menopause. This is likely to be caused by the drop in estrogen, which is vital for protecting against breakages.

Women are also at higher risk of developing osteoporosis as we have smaller bones and have a longer life expectancy, so bone breakdown occurs for longer. Other general risk factors include:

- long-term use of high-dose oral steroids
- a family history of osteoporosis
- long-term use of medications that can affect bone strength or hormone levels

> ### Did you know?
> One in two women and one in five men over the age of 50 experience fractures, mostly as a result of low bone strength.[25]

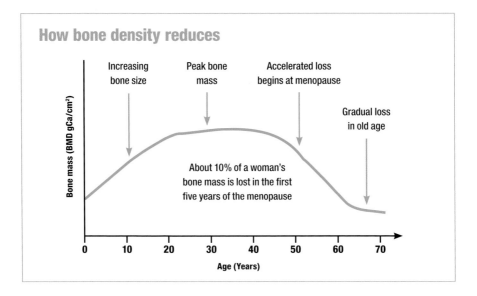

How bone density reduces

Increasing bone size

Peak bone mass

Accelerated loss begins at menopause

Gradual loss in old age

About 10% of a woman's bone mass is lost in the first five years of the menopause

Bone mass (BMD gCa/cm²)

Age (Years)

- a low body mass index
- smoking and heavy drinking.

People with osteoporosis have an increased risk of 'fragility fractures', where normal stresses on your bones from sitting, standing, coughing or even hugging can result in painful fractures. There are usually no outwards signs of osteoporosis, so a broken bone is often the first sign of the condition. These fractures can happen in any of your bones, including your hips, wrists and spine, and can cause pain and even disability.

Cardiovascular disease

Cardiovascular disease refers to conditions affecting the heart and blood vessels – our veins, arteries and capillaries (small blood vessels). Types of cardiovascular disease include coronary heart disease (angina and heart attack), stroke and vascular dementia.

Estrogen protects our arteries in a number of ways, including by reducing the build-up of fatty plaques. Plaques cause the arteries to harden and narrow, so not enough blood and oxygen can get to our vital organs. Because of this, you are at an increased risk of cardiovascular disease during and after your menopause. Low estrogen can also increase cholesterol levels, which can further increase your risk of heart disease. Other general risk factors include:

- being overweight
- high blood pressure
- diabetes
- smoking
- family history of cardiovascular disease.

The increased risk of cardiovascular disease and osteoporosis is far greater if you have an early menopause. A health professional will be able to discuss this with you in more detail, and it is important to know that this increased risk can be reversed with hormone treatment.

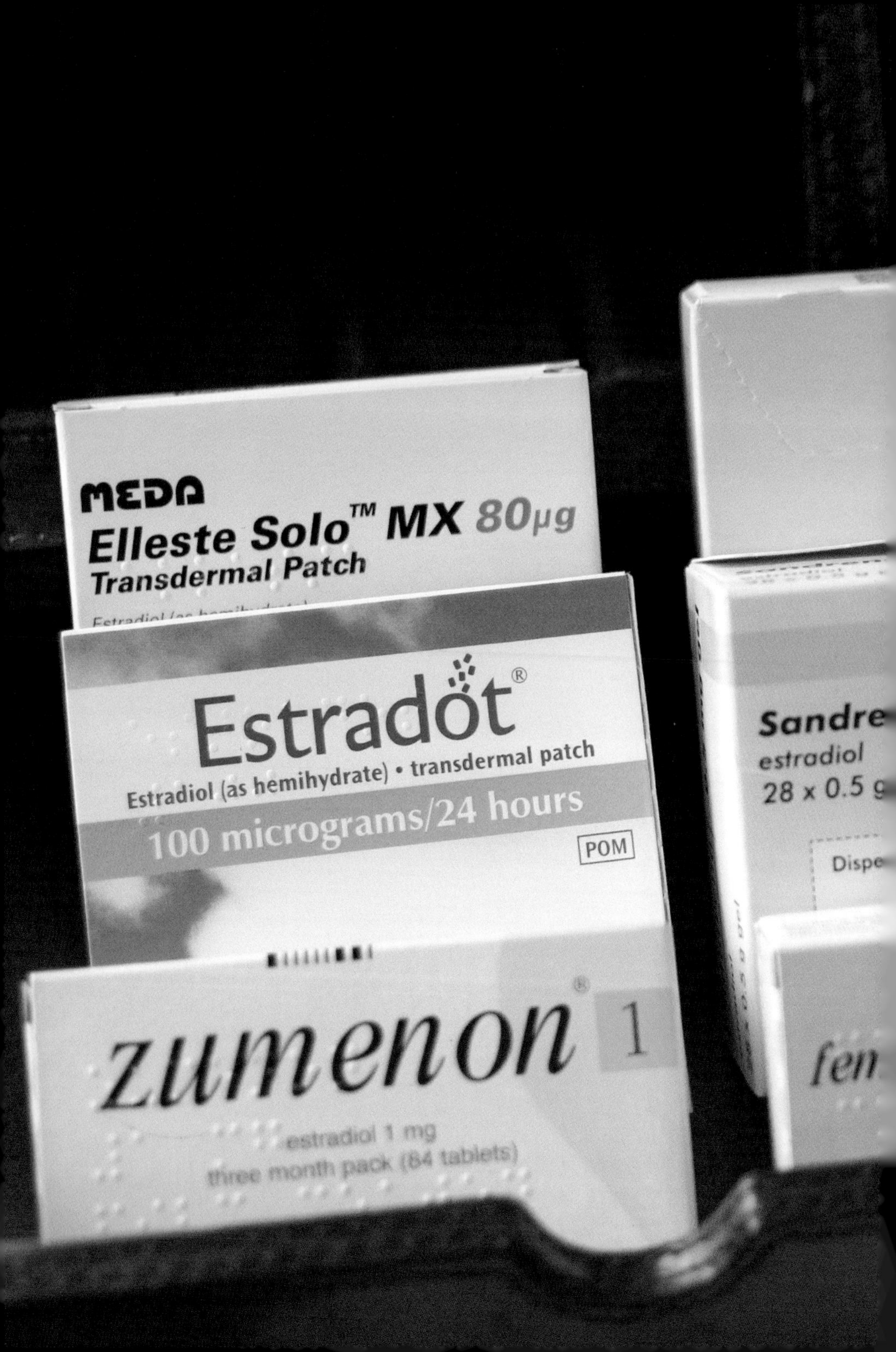

MEDA
Elleste Solo™ MX 80μg
Transdermal Patch

Estradiol (as hemihydrate)

Estradot ®
Estradiol (as hemihydrate) • transdermal patch
100 micrograms/24 hours

POM

zumenon 1

estradiol 1 mg
three month pack (84 tablets)

Sandre
estradiol
28 x 0.5 g

Dispe

fen

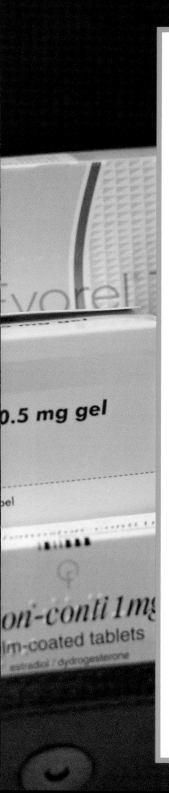

Chapter 3
Time to rethink HRT

Getting the right treatment for your menopausal symptoms can often mean the difference between a miserable menopause and a healthy, manageable one. HRT can have a dramatic effect on your symptoms – many women tell me it literally gives them their life back. Yet, frustratingly, so many others struggle on needlessly for years, despite the fact that HRT is recommended as an effective treatment by medicines watchdog NICE. Why?

Confusion over the safety of HRT, scaremongering headlines and unhelpful myths in recent years have made many women wary of HRT. In this chapter I want to dispel those myths and arm you with the facts to help you make an informed decision on whether HRT is right for you, including:

◆ What HRT actually is
◆ Its benefits and risks
◆ Why you shouldn't wait until your symptoms become unbearable to start treatment.

HRT: What you need to know

Giving HRT to menopausal women is one of the most rewarding things I do as a doctor. Witnessing the transformation of a woman returning to my clinic after taking HRT for three months or so is often remarkable.

Women often tell me how their confidence has soared, their energy levels are amazing, relationships with their partners, friends, families and work colleagues have improved and their joie de vivre has returned.

HRT addresses the underlying cause of your symptoms, protects your bones and safeguards against cardiovascular disease. So in addition to helping you feel better, you can be reassured that taking HRT is actually a real investment for your future health. Yet it is estimated that in some parts of the UK just one in ten menopausal women who would stand to benefit from HRT actually takes it.[1] This means that many women are suffering from menopausal symptoms and increasing their risk of osteoporosis and cardiovascular disease by not taking HRT.

It is time to rethink HRT. Since headlines linking the treatment with breast cancer and blood clots in the early 2000s, the evidence has been re-examined, and new studies carried out. Today, the evidence is clear: for the vast majority of women under the age of 60, the benefits of HRT outweigh any risks.[26]

⬇ HRT tackles symptoms, protects bones and safeguards against cardiovascular disease.

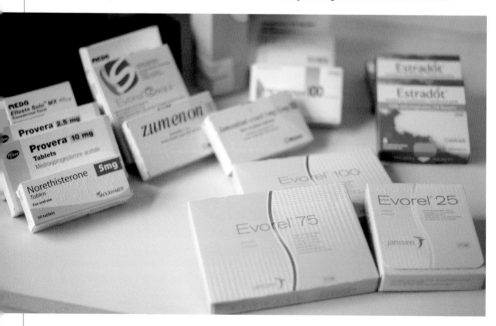

Myths about HRT

MYTH: You should wait until your symptoms become unbearable before starting HRT.

 FALSE: You can start taking HRT as soon as you begin experiencing symptoms, even when you are perimenopausal. There is no need to delay and struggle on. Not only will your immediate symptoms be tackled sooner, there's increasing evidence that the earlier HRT is started, the more it protects you from osteoporosis and cardiovascular disease.

MYTH: You can't take HRT if you suffer from migraines.

 FALSE: If you have a history of migraine, you should opt for HRT in the form of a patch, gel or spray rather than a tablet. Women who have migraines with aura have a small increased risk of stroke which can increase with taking tablet estrogen, but not a patch, gel or spray.

MYTH: You have to stop HRT after five years.

 FALSE: There is no maximum amount of time a woman can take HRT for. You and your doctor need to take into account your individual risks and benefits. Some women take it for a couple of years to help improve their symptoms, others take it for longer – my oldest patient is in her 90s. The vast majority of women starting HRT under 60 years, the benefits of HRT outweigh the risks. Younger women need to take HRT until they are at least 51 years.

MYTH: My menopause will kick in if I stop taking HRT.

 FALSE: HRT doesn't delay your menopause. If your symptoms return when you stop taking HRT this is not an effect of taking hormones, this is because you would still be having symptoms of the menopause at that time if you had never taken it.

MYTH: All HRT causes breast cancer.

 FALSE: HRT containing only estrogen is not associated with an increased risk of breast cancer. Some types of combined HRT may be associated with a small increased risk. Women who take body-identical progesterone do not have an increased risk of breast cancer for the first five years of taking it, and after that it is still debatable whether there really is an increased risk. Women who take older types of progestogens are thought to have a very low risk of breast cancer. This risk of breast cancer with taking HRT is actually lower than the risk of breast cancer in a woman who drinks a couple of glasses of wine most nights, is overweight or who does no exercise.

MYTH: You can't take HRT and vaginal estrogen together.

 FALSE: You can use both together to combat vaginal symptoms such as dryness and other symptoms elsewhere in your body.

Health professionals like myself refer to a number of different guidelines on how we can best help women through their menopause, including guidance from the British Menopause Society and the International Menopause Society. In 2015, guidance on menopause was published by NICE, an independent organisation that decides what drugs and treatments should be made available on the NHS in England. In its first-ever guideline on the menopause, NICE gives clear recommendations on the diagnosis and treatment. It highlights that women whose lives are being affected by the symptoms should not feel they have to suffer in silence.[26]

The guideline makes several recommendations about HRT, including:

◆ HRT is effective for treating several menopausal symptoms, including hot flushes, night sweats and low mood.

◆ If HRT is suitable for you and you are interested in taking it, your doctor should discuss the benefits and risks with you before you decide to start it, both in the short term (the next five years) and in the future.

As you will see in this chapter, HRT is not a one-size-fits-all treatment. It is important that your individual health is taken into account and that the benefits and risks are discussed with your health professional so you have the right type and dosage for you.

So let's take a look at the facts.

What is HRT?

HRT is a treatment that relieves symptoms of your menopause by replacing the estrogen your body stops producing during your menopause. All forms of HRT contain estrogen, which will work to ease symptoms such as hot flushes, mood changes and urinary symptoms.

HRT comes in two types:

◆ **Estrogen only:** the type of estrogen most commonly used nowadays is 17-beta estradiol

◆ **Combined HRT:** this is estrogen (again usually in the form of 17-beta estradiol), plus a version of your hormone progesterone (known as a progestogen if it is synthetic).

Single or combined HRT: what's best for me?

Estrogen-only HRT should only be prescribed if you have had a hysterectomy (have had your uterus removed). If you still have a uterus, it is important that a progestogen is combined with the estrogen. When you take estrogen, the lining of your uterus can build up, which can slightly increase your risk of uterine (womb) cancer. However, taking a progestogen at the same time protects the lining of the uterus and so completely reverses this risk.

➜ HRT can be given in various ways, such as a tablet, patch, gel or spray.

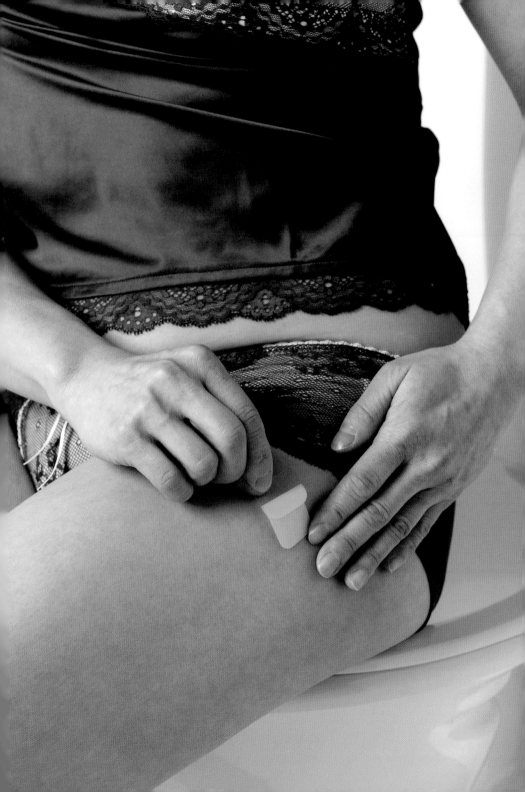

Ways you can take estrogen

Method	How it works	Pros
Oral estrogen tablet	Taken daily	◆ Easy to remember
Estrogen spray	Spray containing replacement estrogen sprayed onto skin, usually on inner forearm or inner thigh	◆ Easily absorbed ◆ Easy to alter dose by increasing/reducing number of sprays under guidance from health professional
Estrogen skin patch	Patches stuck to skin (usually on bottom or upper thigh) and changed twice a week or weekly	◆ Easy to use and stick well to the skin ◆ You can shower, bathe and swim with them on ◆ Constant level given so can be a good option if you get migraines ◆ More than one patch can be used at a time – useful if you have early menopause or POI and may need higher doses of estrogen
Estrogen gel	Gel is rubbed on the arms or legs. It comes in pump packs or sachets. Your doctor or menopause specialist will tell you how much to use	◆ Easy to alter dose so you have more control ◆ Can be used in combination with patches to 'top up' if dose needs to be increased ◆ If you are still having periods it eases premenstrual symptoms (can use more on the days when symptoms are worse)
Estrogen implant	An implant injected under your skin that gradually releases estrogen over several months (this method is far less commonly used)	◆ Can be useful for women who do not absorb estrogen well
Topical vaginal estrogen	Estrogen can be delivered directly to your vagina via a cream, vaginal tablet or ring, to ease symptoms such as dryness	◆ Topical estrogen does not have the same risks associated with it as HRT as it restores estrogen to vagina and surrounding tissues without giving estrogen to whole body ◆ Can be used alongside HRT

Cons

- *I don't usually prescribe first as there is a slight increase in the risk of clots*
- *Less reliable absorption*
- *Oral estrogen can lower your libido further*
- *May not be suitable if you are obese or have conditions like type 2 diabetes or gallbladder disease*
- *If you have early menopause or POI you may need higher doses of estrogen, so might need to use spray in larger quantities*

- *You might not like the sensation of something stuck to your skin*
- *Can lead to local irritation and plaster marks (although marks can be easily removed with baby oil and a dry flannel)*
- *Some women find they don't stick well or they crinkle (therefore reducing absorption)*

- *Absorbs into the skin easily*
- *If you have an early menopause or POI, you often need higher doses, so would need to use large quantities*
- *Sachets can be hard to open if using sachets rather than a pump*

- *Can lead to fluctuating hormone levels*
- *Has to be inserted by specialist doctor so is less flexible*

- *As this is not HRT, it does not improve other symptoms related to the menopause*

How do I take HRT?

HRT comes in about 50 different combinations, with different hormones and doses that can be taken in various ways, such as a tablet, patch, gel or spray (see 'Ways you can take estrogen' table for more information). At first glance it may seem confusing, but the variety available means that the dose and type can be altered to suit your individual needs, in discussion with a health professional. What HRT you can take will depend on your overall health and risk factors for other conditions, for example if you have had a clot in the past or have high blood pressure.

Estrogen is available as a tablet, skin patch, gel, spray or implant. It is also available as a topical cream, vaginal tablet or ring for vaginal and urinary symptoms. Estrogen is often still prescribed in the form of an oral tablet, which evidence suggests can accelerate clotting proteins in the blood. So I usually offer patients the patch, gel or spray, which does not carry a risk of blood clots as the estrogen is absorbed through the skin, rather than affecting the liver which produces our clotting factors.

Progestogen is available as a tablet and also as a coil, which is useful if you are still having periods and need contraception.

Tablets and patches that combine both estrogen and progestogen are also available. I don't usually prescribe these combination products, because there is less flexibility if you want to alter the estrogen dose. Combined HRT also contains older progestogens.

For my patients who need a progestogen, I usually prescribe a newer type called micronised progesterone, derived from yams, the tropical root vegetable. Some studies show that

Ways you can take progestogen

Method	How it works	Pros
Micronised progesterone	Taken as a tablet	◆ Has fewer side effects than other types of progestogen ◆ Some studies show a lower risk of breast cancer than other progestogens ◆ Often has mild sedation as a side effect which many women find beneficial
Intrauterine system (IUS) or coil	A small, T-shaped plastic device is inserted into your uterus by a doctor or nurse, which releases progestogen at a constant rate	◆ Provides a form of contraception for women who still need it ◆ Less risk of bleeding ◆ Can stay in place for up to five years

micronised progesterone is associated with a lower risk of breast cancer, cardiovascular disease and clots than older progestogens. I also often recommend the progestogen-containing coil.

If you have a history of clot, migraine, diabetes or liver disease you can still take HRT but it is likely that you will be recommended to use an estrogen patch, gel or spray as it is associated with fewer risks than a tablet. If you also need progestogen, then this is usually still given as a tablet or the progestogen-containing coil.

I need combined HRT: how often do I take it?

How you take combined HRT depends on whether you are still having periods. If you are still having regular periods, you should take cyclical HRT, which still give

Combined HRT at a glance

Type of HRT	Bleeding frequency	Best for	Progestogen taken
Cyclical monthly	Every month	If you still have monthly periods	10–14 days each month
Cyclical 3-monthly	14 days every 13 weeks	Irregular periods	14 days every three months
Continuous	None	If your periods have stopped	Every day

- ◆ Can cause breakthrough bleeding in the first few months
- ◆ Needs to be taken on an empty stomach
- ◆ Not a contraceptive, but if a woman has no period for a year with taking micronised progesterone then it can be considered a contraceptive

- ◆ Can lead to spotting in the first 3–6 months after insertion
- ◆ Not always available in primary care
- ◆ Contains an older type of progestogen

you a regular bleed. This bleed is not a period, rather the progestogen causing the lining of the uterus to shed. This type of HRT needs to be taken for about a year, as if you use continuous HRT too soon it can lead to very irregular periods. There are two types of cyclical HRT:

1 Monthly, where you take estrogen every day, and then progestogen at the end of the month for a set number of days. This is best if you are still having monthly periods.
2 Three-monthly: you take estrogen every day and progestogen for a set number of days every three months, giving you a bleed every three months. This is best if you have irregular periods.

My periods have stopped: what should I take?
If you haven't had a period for a year, its likely you will be given a type of HRT

Bleeding and continuous HRT

It is completely normal to experience some spotting or light bleeding in the first few months of taking this type of HRT. However, if you experience prolonged vaginal bleeding you should let your health professional know.

which doesn't cause a monthly bleed, called continuous combined HRT. As the name suggests, both estrogen and progestogen are taken every day, usually without a break.

Relief at last: what will happen to my symptoms?
Many women find that many of their symptoms of the menopause improve within a few months of taking HRT. They often notice that their sleep, mood and concentration improve, their energy levels recover and their skin and hair look healthier.

Hot flushes and night sweats usually stop within a few weeks, while vaginal and urinary symptoms – such as dryness, discomfort during sex, recurrent urine infections and increased urination – should improve within one to three months. However, it can take up to a year for some women.

It is very common for the dose and sometimes the type of HRT to be altered if you are still having symptoms after you have been taking HRT for a few months. Some women find their symptoms initially improve then worsen, and this is usually due to them having inadequate estrogen.

Let's talk about the benefits

In addition to providing much-needed relief from your symptoms, HRT can have several benefits.

Your cardiovascular disease risk will reduce

HRT does not increase your risk of heart disease when it is started if you are under 60 years.[26] There is plenty of evidence that taking HRT actually reduces your risk of developing cardiovascular disease. The benefits are greatest in those women who start HRT within ten years of their menopause.[27] High cholesterol is another risk factor for cardiovascular disease, and HRT can help to lower cholesterol levels.[28]

Your risk of developing osteoporosis will reduce

Taking HRT can prevent and reverse the bone loss that occurs, even for those women who take low doses of HRT. This means that taking HRT reduces your risk of having a fracture due to osteoporosis.[26] Even low doses of estrogen can offer bone protection.

Other possible benefits

Some studies have shown a reduced risk of developing Alzheimer's disease and other types of dementia in women who take HRT. In addition, some studies have also shown a reduction in risk of bowel cancer in women who take HRT. Studies have also shown there is a reduction in risk of type 2 diabetes and also osteoarthritis.

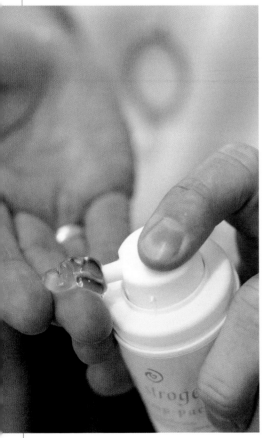

⬈ TV presenter and journalist Lorraine Kelly has been so supportive of my work. She has really helped break down the taboo around menopause by speaking candidly about her own menopause experience and how HRT has helped her symptoms

⬅ Estrogen, when applied as a gel, is safe and effective.

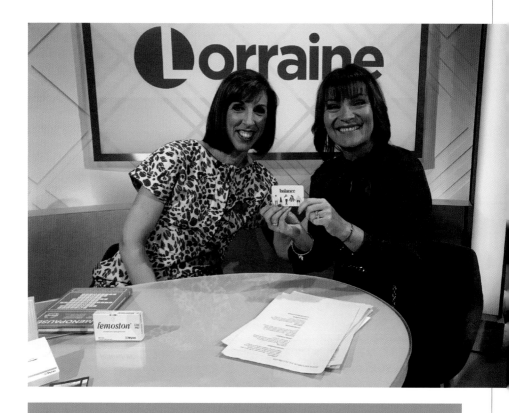

HRT: my experience

As I am otherwise fit and healthy, I decided that HRT was the best option for me to help my perimenopausal symptoms, which had been having a very negative impact on the quality of my life. I started taking HRT in 2017 and, while my husband was supportive of my decision, the reaction from some of my friends was surprising, with comments including: 'Surely you are too young for HRT.' (I was 46 at the time I started taking it – and there's no age restriction to taking HRT.) 'But HRT is so dangerous.' (As we know, the benefits of HRT outweigh the risks in the vast majority of women under 60 years of age.)

But for me, deciding to take HRT was the best move I could have made, both for my physical health and for my wellbeing. Once my preparations and dosages were adjusted after the first few months, I felt amazing – my energy levels were better than they had been for decades, I was able to multitask again and my concentration was so much better. My skin and hair looked healthier and my joints didn't feel as stiff when I did yoga. Such was the positive change in me that my husband remarked that he wished he could take a male type of HRT.

Let's talk about the risks

HRT has been available in the UK since the 1960s. In 2002, the Women's Health Initiative study voiced concerns of an increased risk of breast cancer, some increased risk of cardiovascular disease, and more harm than benefit overall in women who took combined HRT.[29]

However, it is very important to look at the design of this study. The women in this study were on average 63 years old, which means that they no longer had menopausal symptoms. Also, many of the women were overweight or obese and had also had heart attacks in the past. All the women in the study were given oral estrogen and an older type of progestogen as their HRT. This means that these women already had other risk factors for heart disease and cancer. Yet much of the media hype that surrounded the study failed to highlight these facts, and the findings sparked huge concerns among doctors and women.

Thankfully, things have moved on. The original Women's Health Initiative data have been re-examined and further studies have been conducted that show that for most women who start taking HRT when they are under 60, the benefits of HRT outweigh the risks. In addition, the types of HRT used in this study are not the types commonly used now.

Your actual risk of developing the diseases mentioned here depends on many factors, such as your age, family history and general health, and not solely on whether or not you take HRT. This is why is it crucial for your doctor to discuss your individual risks and benefits of taking HRT. You can greatly reduce your risk of developing heart disease, stroke and many cancers through key lifestyle changes such as not smoking, taking regular exercise and eating a healthy diet – more of which in the next chapter.

Breast cancer

In my experience, breast cancer is the risk that most women worry about with HRT and the one that women will ask me about first. Here is what you need to know.

1 Overall, one in eight women will develop breast cancer in their lifetime.[30] Each woman's risk of developing breast cancer is different, and is down to different factors including their age, genetics and lifestyle.

2 There is no increased risk of breast cancer in women who take HRT under the age of 51 years.

3 If you are only taking estrogen-only HRT then studies have shown that there is no increased risk of breast cancer.

4 Taking some types of combined HRT may be associated with a small increased risk of developing breast cancer.

5 This risk increases the longer you use combined HRT. When you stop taking combined HRT, you have the same risk of breast cancer as someone who has never taken HRT.

6 There has never been a study which has shown there's an increased risk of dying from breast cancer in women who take HRT.

7 Observational studies have shown that micronised progesterone may be

associated with a lower risk of breast cancer than other progestogens for the first five years.

Clots in the veins (venous thromboembolism)

When blood moves too slowly around the body, it can cause blood cells to clump together in a clot. When a clot forms in a vein deep inside your body, it is called a deep vein thrombosis (or DVT). In some women, this clot may travel to your lung and cause a pulmonary embolism. Together, DVT and pulmonary embolism are known as venous thromboembolism.

Women who take combined HRT as tablets have an increased risk of developing a clot. This is because taking estrogen as a tablet activates the factors in the liver that clot your blood. This does not happen when the estrogen is used as a patch, gel or spray.

You are more likely to develop a clot if you have other risk factors. These include being obese, having a clot in the past and being a smoker. However, the risk of getting a clot is still very low in most women. This risk of clot is not present in women who use patches, gels or sprays rather than HRT tablets. This is because HRT is absorbed directly into the bloodstream and doesn't have to be processed by the liver, so there is no increased risk of clots.

Stroke

While the risk of stroke for women under 60 years is very low,[26] some studies have shown that there is a small increased risk of stroke in women taking either estrogen alone or combined HRT as tablets.

Some risks of HRT, such as blood clots and stroke, are higher with oral estrogen (although the overall risk is still small). However, there is no increased risk of stroke in women who use the patch, gel or spray rather than tablets. In addition, oral HRT containing lower doses of estrogen seems to be associated with a lower risk of stroke than those containing higher doses.

What side effects can I expect?

Side effects are more likely to occur when you first start taking HRT and then they usually settle with time.

The most common side effects in the first few weeks of taking HRT are irregular bleeding, some breast discomfort or leg cramps. These tend to go within a few months if you continue to take HRT. Some women find that certain makes of skin patches irritate their skin. A change to a different brand or type of HRT may help if this happens.

Various estrogens and progestogens are used in the different brands. If you have a side effect with one brand, it may not happen with a different one. Changing the delivery method of HRT (for example, from a tablet to a patch) may also help to reduce side effects.

HIV and menopause

Advances in medication mean that, thankfully, HIV is now seen as a long-term, manageable. According to the NHS, with an early diagnosis and effective treatments, most people with HIV will not develop any AIDS-related illnesses and will live a near-normal expectancy[31a].

According to one study, in 2016, 10,350 women living with HIV aged between 45 and 56 (potentially menopausal age) attended for HIV care in the UK; a five-fold increase over ten years[31b].

◆ **What sort of symptoms can I expect?**
You may be affected by any of the symptoms listed in chapter 2. The PRIME study, which looked at the health and well-being of 900 women aged 45-60-year-olds living with HIV, found well-being of women living with HIV found a high prevalence of symptoms such as hot flushes, muscle and joint pains and sleep disturbance.

Nine out of ten women reported urogenital symptoms (such as vaginal dryness and urinary symptoms), and 78% of women reported psychological symptoms such as anxiety, low mood and irritability.

◆ **Long-term health implications**
People living with HIV have a greater incidence of bone mineral density loss and fragility fractures. According to the Terrance Higgins Trust, opinion is divided on whether this is because of the virus itself, side effects of treatment or inflammation [source https://www.tht.org.uk/hiv-and-sexual-health/living-hiv-long-term/osteoporosis]

◆ **Can I take HRT if I am living with HIV?**
Yes. However, the PRIME study shows too few women living with HIV receive HRT– just 8% of women with HIV told the PRIME study they were taking hormone replacement therapy. If you feel you aren't getting the correct advice, ask to be referred to a menopause specialist.

◆ **Where should I go for further advice?**
Good online sources of advice include the Terrance Higgins Trust (www.tht.org.uk) as well as NAM, a UK charity which shares information about HIV and AIDS (www.aidsmap.com)

The truth about HRT

Researcher, writer and broadcaster Liz Earle MBE works tremendously hard to bust myths about the menopause in the media, and has been a mentor and real inspiration to to me. Her e-book, the Truth about HRT, is essential reading (www. lizearlewellbeing.com).

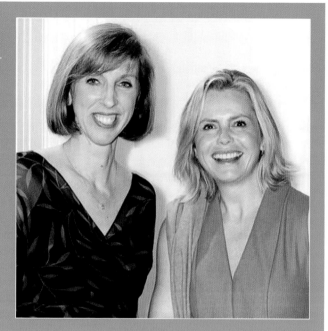

Does HRT mean I don't need contraception?

HRT contains low levels of hormones and so does not work as a contraception. If you still require contraception, then you should talk to your doctor about the options available to you. The only exception would be if you are using an IUS (intrauterine system) or coil for the progestogen element of your HRT as this also acts as a contraceptive.

If you have POI

If you have a premature menopause (POI, see Chapter 1), you should take hormones (either HRT or the combined oral contraceptive pill) until at least the natural age of menopause, so around 51 years of age. This will be simply replacing hormones that your body would otherwise be making up to the age of natural menopause. It will not only improve your menopausal symptoms, but it is vital for your future health to safeguard against an increased risk of osteoporosis and cardiovascular disease.

Any risks of HRT don't apply if you have POI and are taking HRT.[32]

POI can be a devastating diagnosis for some women, and many women find that they experience anxiety or even depression after being diagnosed with POI. You should not be ashamed if you have these symptoms. It is really important to talk about any symptoms you may be experiencing as there's effective treatment available to help you.

You can ask about a referral to a specialist menopause clinic. The Daisy Network is a charity dedicated to providing information and support for women and girls diagnosed with POI (www.daisynetwork.org.uk).

Body-identical or bioidentical HRT: what you need to know

It is understandable that many women would prefer to take natural products to tackle their menopausal symptoms, but 'natural' doesn't necessarily mean something is safer or better for you. You may have heard about more modern preparations of HRT known as body-identical HRT and bioidentical HRT. They sound similar, but there are crucial differences, outlined below.

Body-identical HRT

Some older types of HRT contain a mixture of different types of estrogens and are made from pregnant mare's urine. While this estrogen comes from a natural source, it is not identical to the estrogen we want to replace in our bodies, and so this type of HRT contains many types of estrogens we don't need.

Nowadays another type of estrogen is available on the NHS and through menopause specialists like me, known as body-identical estrogen. This means it has the same molecular structure as the estrogen that decreases in your body during your menopause. It is extracted from the yam, a tropical root vegetable. Some types of body-identical estrogens (such as 17 beta oestradiol, which I usually prescribe for women) are available on the NHS and through menopause specialists in the form of patches, gels or sprays.

Likewise, a type of body-identical progestogen can also usually be prescribed on the NHS and by menopause specialists. The type of progestogen I commonly prescribe for my patients is called micronised progesterone, which is also derived from yams. Micronised progesterone is associated with fewer side effects than other types of progestogens,

which can include bloating, spots and mood swings. Studies show that micronised progesterone is not associated with an increased risk of breast cancer for the first five years of taking it. After this time, the risks of breast cancer are very low and seem to be lower than the risk for a woman taking the older types of progestogen.[33]

So, in summary, body-identical hormones:

◆ have the same molecular structure as the hormones in our body
◆ are usually available on the NHS and privately
◆ and, crucially, have been tested, regulated and deemed safe to use.

Bioidentical hormones

Bioidentical hormones are like body-identical hormones in that they are made from plant sources, but the similarities end there. Bioidentical hormones are not available on the NHS. Instead, some private clinics offer bioidentical treatment that is 'compounded' or custom-made to suit your individual hormone levels following various blood or saliva tests.

These treatments have not been subjected to the same tests of safety, efficacy or dosing consistency as the HRT prescribed on the NHS or by someone like myself. There is no good evidence to suggest that compounded bioidentical hormones are more effective or have fewer side effects than conventional HRT. I see women in my clinic who have spent considerable amounts of money on these bioidentical products and have experienced numerous side effects. The products used in this way are not regulated or approved and so could potentially be harmful.

The British Menopause Society's position on bioidentical HRT is clear: bioidentical products are not recommended because they are not regulated and not evidence based for effectiveness and safety. It adds that

Natural progesterone creams?

You may see 'natural' progesterone skin creams advertised online. They are not recommended as they don't absorb into the body well and many contain amounts of hormone that are too small to be effective.

there is insufficient evidence to justify the multiple serum and salivary hormone tests often claimed to precisely individualise treatment.[34]

⬇ Body-identical HRT is derived from the yam which is a root vegetable.

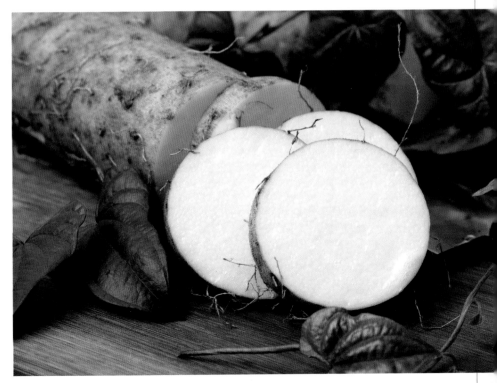

Testosterone

Testosterone helps to regulate sex drive and has a role to play in energy levels and bone and brain health. Levels of testosterone can fall during and after your menopause. In fact, women produce three times as much testosterone than estrogen before their menopause.

Do I need testosterone?

Not all women will need testosterone to help ease their menopausal symptoms. However, if you find that HRT alone is not effective in improving your sex drive and other symptoms such as mood and concentration, then a testosterone supplement can be prescribed to restore your testosterone levels back to levels before your menopause. NICE recommends that doctors can prescribe testosterone for menopausal women with low sex drive if HRT alone is not effective.[26]

Loss of testosterone can be quite noticeable if you have a surgical menopause, or have POI (see Chapter 1), when testosterone production decreases by more than 50%.[35]

Testosterone is usually only prescribed by a doctor who specialises in the menopause because the use of testosterone for low sex drive in women is currently unlicensed in the UK. This does not mean that it is unsafe, rather that the manufacturer of the treatment has not specified that it can be used in this way.

How do I take it?

Testosterone is usually given as a cream or gel that you rub into your skin (usually on your lower abdomen or outer thigh) so it goes directly into your bloodstream. Alternatively, testosterone may be given to some women as an implant.

How long will it take to work?

It can sometimes take a few months for the full effects of testosterone to work in your body. Although it may not be effective for every woman, for some it really can make a huge difference. Younger women who have had an early menopause often notice benefits from using testosterone.

Are there any side effects/risks?

There are usually no side effects with testosterone treatment as it is given to replace the testosterone that you are otherwise lacking. Very occasionally, women notice some increased hair growth in the area into which they have rubbed the cream.[35] You can avoid this by changing the area of skin on which you rub the cream.

→ Testosterone can be prescribed for low sex drive if HRT alone is not effective.

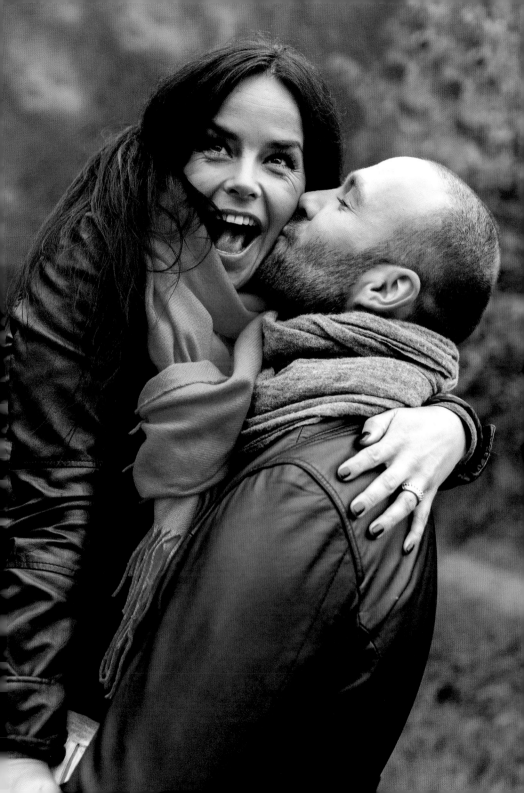

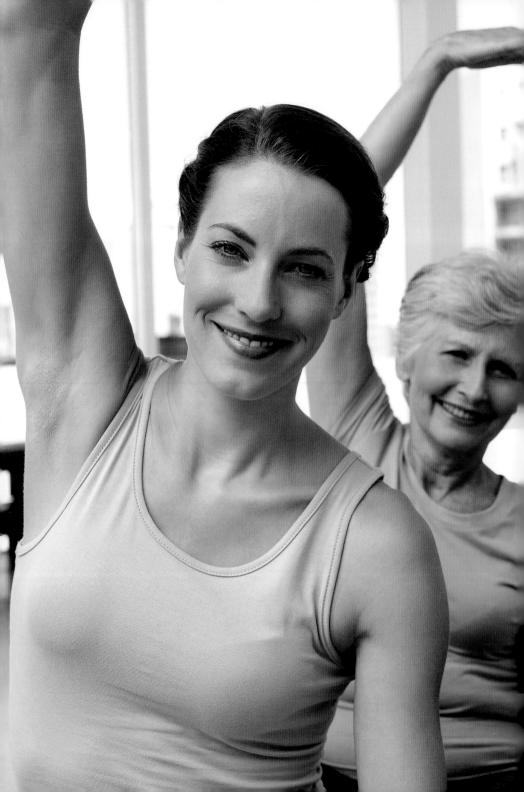

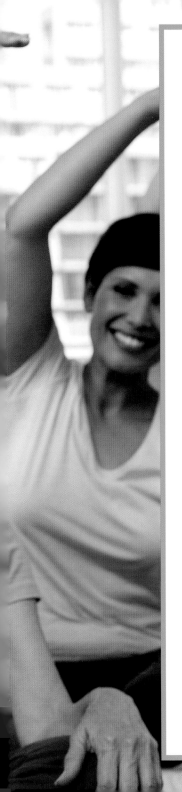

Chapter 4
Alternative treatments and lifestyle changes

Although HRT remains the first-line treatment for menopausal symptoms for most women, you might not be able to take it for medical reasons, or you might choose not to take it. And even if you do take HRT, there is so much more to menopause management than simply just prescribing HRT. It is essential at this time to take a holistic approach to your menopause and life in general. As well as making sure you are taking the right balance and strength of hormones for you, you should be optimising your nutrition, exercise, sleep and wellbeing. This chapter looks at the range of alternative treatments available, including:

◆ Non-hormonal treatments
◆ Cognitive behavioural therapy
◆ Herbal medicines, and why 'natural' might not always mean better for you
◆ Holistic approaches, including yoga
◆ A healthier, happier you: how diet, exercise and lifestyle changes lay the foundation for a healthier menopause.

Prescription non-hormonal treatments

There are some non-hormonal treatments available on prescription that can help with symptoms such as hot flushes and night sweats, low mood, anxiety and also vaginal dryness. These treatments might not be suitable for everyone, and their side effects can limit use, so discuss them with your health professional before you decide to take them.

Antidepressants

Certain types of antidepressants such as citalopram or venlafaxine in low doses can reduce hot flushes and night sweats in some women. They are often offered and given to women who have a history of breast cancer. They can start to improve symptoms within a few days or weeks. Side effects can include a dry mouth, constipation and reduced libido in some women.

If you are being offered antidepressants by your health professional, be sure to clarify exactly what symptoms they are being prescribed for. Although antidepressants can help with vasomotor symptoms (hot flushes and night sweats)

⬇ There are alternative medications available for women who can not take HRT for medical reasons or who chose not to take HRT.

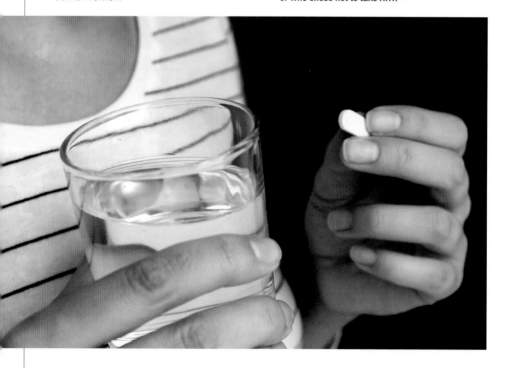

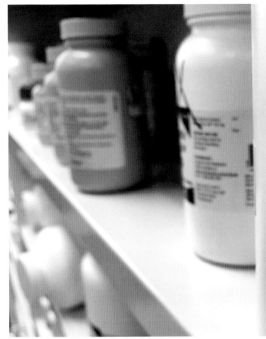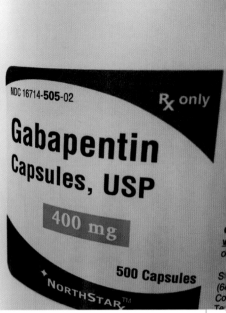

↑ Gabapentin may be used for hot flushes, but does have side effects such as drowsiness and dizziness.

many women are incorrectly prescribed them for menopause-related mood changes and they do not usually help for these.

My recent survey of almost 3,000 women found that nearly two-thirds were given antidepressants for menopause-related low mood rather than HRT. The NICE guidelines make it clear: there is no actual evidence that antidepressants ease low mood in menopausal women who have not been diagnosed with clinical depression.[26]

Clonidine

Clonidine is a medication mainly used to treat high blood pressure, but it is also the only non-hormone treatment licensed to treat hot flushes in the UK. However, in my experience it does not usually work and its use is often limited by side effects such as nausea, low blood pressure, and dry mouth. NICE menopause guidelines recommend that antidepressants and clonidine should not be used as first treatment just for vasomotor symptoms.[26]

Gabapentin

Gabapentin is a medication that is usually used to treat epilepsy, but it can reduce hot flushes in some women after a few weeks. The NICE menopause guidelines do not specifically mention gabapentin, but International Menopause Society guidelines state that it can be effective like antidepressants, but this medication can have side effects such as drowsiness and dizziness.[36]

Cognitive behavioural therapy

If you are finding mood changes hard to cope with, then your health professional may suggest trying Cognitive Behavioural Therapy (or CBT). According to the mental health charity Mind, CBT is a talking treatment that focuses on how your thoughts, beliefs and attitudes affect your feelings and behaviour, and teaches you coping skills for dealing with different problems.[37]

CBT address problems by helping to change the way you think (cognitive) and how you act (behaviour) and is commonly used for anxiety and depression, as well as for phobias and sleep problems. It has also been shown to help with menopausal symptoms, and NICE recommends that it can help to alleviate menopause-related low mood or anxiety.[26] According to a review published in the International Journal of Obstetrics and Gynaecology, psychological interventions such as CBT and mindfulness can help women suffering from hot flushes and other symptoms like irritability, forgetfulness, joint pain and vaginal dryness.[38]

How does it work?

CBT is delivered by a trained therapist either one on one or as part of a group. It focuses on the present, rather than past events, and teaches coping methods to combat negative thoughts and behaviours. You will be asked to break down issues

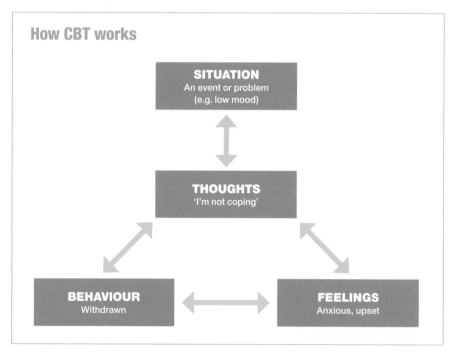

How CBT works

SITUATION
An event or problem
(e.g. low mood)

THOUGHTS
'I'm not coping'

BEHAVIOUR
Withdrawn

FEELINGS
Anxious, upset

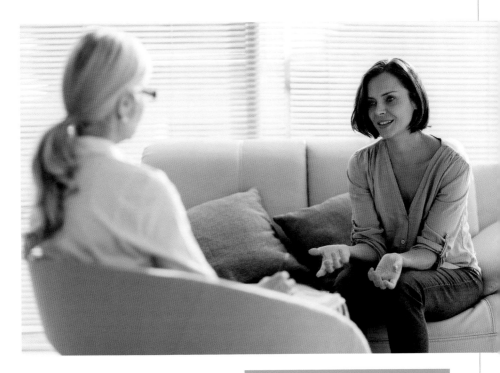

into more manageable parts, typically, situation, thoughts, feelings and behaviour.

During your sessions, you will learn how to recognise how each area impacts on the other – the way you think about a situation influences how your body reacts, how you feel and what you do about it.

How do I get started?

You can self-refer for CBT on the NHS through your local psychological therapies service, or you can ask your GP to refer you. Waiting times can be long and many women find it is quicker to organise help privately.

Are there any risks?

No. You can do CBT alongside other treatments. It will involve doing some 'homework' or exercises outside of your sessions.

For more information

NHS Choices gives information about CBT, including how to find a psychological therapist: www.nhs.uk/conditions/cognitive-behavioural-therapy-cbt

The British Association for Behavioural and Cognitive Psychotherapies keeps a list of CBT therapists accredited by them: www.cbtregisteruk.com

Women's Health Concern, the patient arm of the British Menopause Society, has a good (free) factsheet on CBT and the menopause: www.womens-health-concern.org/help-and-advice/factsheets/cognitive-behaviour-therapy-cbt-menopausal-symptoms

Complementary and alternative medicines

You may be considering some of the complementary or alternative therapies below either on their own (alternative therapy) or alongside conventional treatments (complementary).

These preparations are not usually available on the NHS, so you will probably have to see a private practitioner. It is important to tell your doctor or menopause expert if you are trying a therapy or are taking herbal medicines bought over the counter or prescribed by a herbalist.

Herbal medicines

There is a huge herbal medicines market and a number of preparations that claim to help menopausal symptoms like hot flushes, such as red clover, black cohosh and St John's wort. A word of caution here. Just because a product is 'natural', it does not necessarily mean that it is safer or better for you compared to conventional medicines. Scientific evidence on how effective a herbal medicine is tends to be quite limited.

Potency can vary between products and, like conventional medicine, herbal

Herbal medicines at a glance

Medicine	What is it?	
St John's wort	A flowering plant.	
Black cohosh	A herb in the same plant family as the buttercup.	
Isoflavones	Isoflavones are a type of phytoestrogens, which are compounds similar to the estrogen we produce. Isoflavones and phytoestrogens are found in red clover and also present in very small amounts in foods including soy, flax seeds, lentils and oats.	

medicines can have significant side effects or can interfere with other medicines you might be taking. It is also worth remembering that although some preparations may help with your menopausal symptoms, they won't address your low levels of hormones, improve bone strength or reduce your risk of cardiovascular disease.

Look out for the logo

You should always discuss with a health professional first before taking herbal medicines. If you do decide to try over-the-counter products, look for ones with the Traditional Herbal Registration (THR) marking on the packaging.

The THR is a scheme overseen by the Medicines and Healthcare products Regulatory Agency (or MHRA), the UK

body responsible for ensuring that medicines work and are safe. The mark means the herbal medicine complies with quality standards relating to safety and manufacturing, and it provides information about how and when to use it.[39]

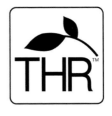

Acupuncture

Acupuncture involves inserting fine needles at specific points in the body. Those who practice the traditional Chinese method of acupuncture believe that it restores the body's 'Qi', or energy flow. Western medical acupuncture uses the needles to stimulate the nervous system and is mainly used to treat musculoskeletal pain.[40]

What is it used for?	NICE's verdict
St John's wort is probably best known as a remedy for depression, but is taken by some women for hot flushes.	*The NICE menopause guideline notes that while St John's wort can reduce hot flushes and night sweats for some women, the ingredients of products containing St John's wort can vary and their effects are uncertain. It also cautions that products can interfere with other drugs, including those used to treat breast cancer (such as tamoxifen).*
It is used by some women for hot flushes and night sweats.	*While there is some evidence that black cohosh may relieve vasomotor symptoms, multiple preparations are available, and their safety is uncertain. Interactions with other medicines have been reported.*
Some women take isoflavones to improve hot flushes and night sweats. Isoflavones as supplements are generally not recommended if you have a history of breast cancer.	*While there is some evidence that isoflavones may relieve vasomotor symptoms, multiple preparations are available, and their safety is uncertain. Interactions with other medicines have been reported.*

Alternate nostril breathing

Alternate nostril breathing (or *nadi shodhana*) is a breathing technique commonly used at the beginning or end of yoga practice. Hillary Clinton has talked about how alternate nostril breathing helped bring about inner calm after the 2016 US election.[42] It's a nice exercise to try at the end of a hectic day to help clear your mind, and is especially useful to relax you if you have trouble sleeping.

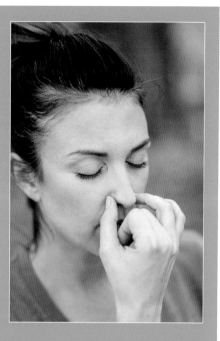

1   Sit tall in a chair or crossed legged on the floor in a quiet room (closing your eyes if you wish).
2   Practise a few long breaths breathing in and out through your nostrils.
3   Place your left hand on your left knee and bring your right hand up towards your face.
4   Exhale completely and use your right thumb to gently close your right nostril.
5   Inhale through your left nostril and use your right ring finger to close your left nostril.
6   Open your right nostril again and exhale.
7   Inhale through your right nostril, then close the nostril again.
8   Open your left nostril and exhale.
9   Repeat for a few minutes each morning and evening.

At present, NICE only recommends acupuncture as a treatment for migraines and chronic headaches, and while there is little scientific evidence to support its use in alleviating menopausal symptoms, some women who use acupuncture have reported some success. Some of my patients have found acupuncture really beneficial so it may be worth considering if you are suffering and not able to take HRT.

Aromatherapy

Aromatherapy is a complementary therapy which uses oils extracted from plants to promote relaxation and wellbeing. These essential oils, such as lavender and rosemary, can be diluted with a carrier oil and absorbed through the skin during massage, inhaled or a few drops can be added to warm bath water.

Although little is known about the effect of aromatherapy on menopausal symptoms,[41] women have told me that they have used oils like lavender to relax and de-stress. I actually use a combination of frankincense and rosemary oils in a pot of hot water when I do yoga and the smell is wonderful and uplifting! Essential oils are very concentrated and may not be suitable for everyone, so do speak to an aromatherapist if you are unsure.

Yoga

Yoga is a mind and body practice that combines physical movements (known as postures), breathing and meditation. Yoga is a fantastic exercise for the entire body. It can also improve some of the symptoms of the menopause, including sleep disturbance, fatigue, low mood and anxiety. Our muscle tone and bone density reduce during the perimenopause and menopause so doing regular yoga practice can also be beneficial for these. Some women find it helps reduce hot flushes too.

Regular yoga practice can help strengthen muscles, improve flexibility and reduce aches and pains, and can also relieve stress and anxiety. I use yoga as part of my own menopause treatment. It stretches and flexes my muscles and brings mental clarity and focus. In fact, we have a yoga studio at my clinic, which many women love and really benefit from.

Petra Coveney is an experienced yoga teacher, who is also a member of the British Menopause Society. After going through her own menopause, Petra developed Menopause Yoga to help other women manage their symptoms.

Menopause Yoga combines western medical science with eastern wellbeing, and includes specially adapted yoga poses, breathing exercises and mindful meditation techniques designed to help women manage some of the main menopause symptoms such as hot flushes, anger surges, anxiety, insomnia, fatigue and low mood.

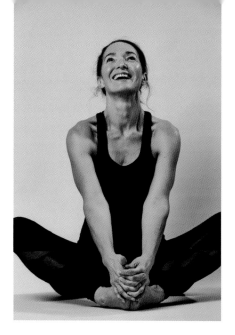

↑ Petra Coveney teaches Menopause Yoga

For more information

Complementary and alternative therapies are not usually available on the NHS and are not subject to professional statutory regulation in the same way as conventional medicine (www.nhs.uk/conditions/complementary-and-alternative-medicine). However, some therapies operate registers that practitioners can apply to join provided they meet criteria such as qualifications and practice standards. These include the:

British Acupuncture Council: www.acupuncture.org.uk

Complementary and Natural Healthcare Council: www.cnhc.org.uk

International Federation of Professional Aromatherapists: www.ifparoma.org

Lifestyle changes: exercise

Getting plenty of exercise can help with the changes your body goes through during your menopause, not to mention your general health and wellbeing. Yet an estimated 40% of adult women in the UK aren't getting enough exercise, putting them at risk of a raft of health problems including type 2 diabetes, cardiovascular disease and cancer.[43]

It is understandable that exercise is probably the last thing on your mind when you have been awake for most of the night, your joints ache or your changing body shape makes you feel self-conscious. But the benefits of exercise are just too important to miss out on – and here's why.

Why is exercise so important during the perimenopause/menopause?

1. For your bone health

Bone breakdown occurs more rapidly than bone build-up during the perimenopause and menopause, and we lose about 10% of our bone mass in the first five years of the menopause. If you are taking HRT, it will help to protect your bones by replacing estrogen. But if you aren't (and even if you are) exercise plays a part too. That's because bone is a living tissue that grows stronger in reaction to increases in loads and forces – which happens when we exercise.

2. For your muscles

We lose muscle mass as we get older, leaving us at risk of falls and fractures, but the good news is that regular exercise can slow this down.

3. For cardiovascular health

You are put at an increased risk of cardiovascular disease during and after your menopause. Regular exercise helps maintain healthy cholesterol and reduces the risk of high blood pressure and cardiovascular disease.[44]

4. For your mood changes

When we exercise, we release feel-good chemicals called endorphins, and activities like yoga can help you to de-stress.

5. To help maintain a healthy weight

Falling estrogen levels can lead to a greater fat distribution around your middle, which increases the risk of cardiovascular disease, diabetes and cancer. Regular exercise and a balanced diet can help.

Stub it out

We all know that smoking is bad news for our general health and raises the risk of cancer, cardiovascular disease and osteoporosis. But did you know studies show smoking can increase the severity and duration of hot flushes, and even suggest an association between smoking and an early menopause? Get help quitting at www.nhs.uk/smokefree.

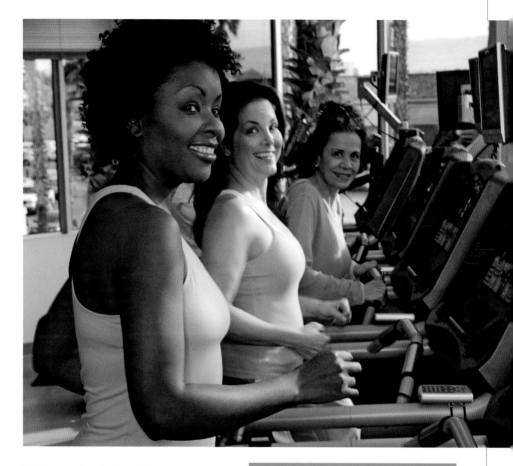

Will exercise help with my hot flushes?

A 2014 review found insufficient evidence to show whether exercise is an effective treatment for vasomotor symptoms (hot flushes and night sweats).[45] However, the numerous benefits of exercise mean that it is still important for your general health.

A 2016 study of 6,000 Latin American women aged 40–59 found that those who had more sedentary lifestyles were more likely to experience severe menopausal symptoms than physically active women, such as vasomotor symptoms, anxiety and sleep disturbance.[46]

How much exercise should I be getting?

Guidelines state that adults between 19 and 64 should be aiming for:

30 minutes of moderate intensity exercise five times a week

plus

strength exercises on two or more days a week.[47]

What types of exercise are good for me?

There are broadly two types of exercise that are good for bone health and will be of particular benefit during this time.

1 Weight-bearing exercises that use your feet and legs to support your weight, including:

◆ brisk walking, jogging or running
◆ dancing
◆ aerobics
◆ badminton or tennis.

Keep your cool

Think thin layers rather than one heavy one when exercising. Look for fabrics from natural fibres like cotton and bamboo, which help wick away sweat.

⬇ Lucy Holtom (pictured) is the main yoga teacher at Newson Health.

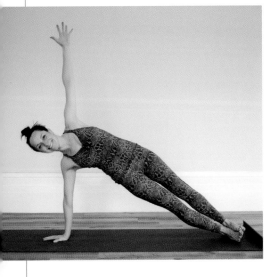

2 Strength exercises using your muscles to pull on your bones, which will boost bone strength, including:

◆ press-ups
◆ using weights or exercise resistance bands
◆ yoga
◆ pilates.

I haven't exercised in a while: where do I start?

The earlier you start, the sooner you will see the benefits. You may find it easier to get into exercise good habits while you are perimenopausal (or even better, before). That's because you may find that once you are menopausal you have less energy or have more physical aches and pains. Doing something is better than nothing at all. Walking is a great way to start, even if just for a few minutes a day.

You could also build some exercise into your daily routine by making some small changes, such as taking the stairs instead of a lift, parking your car slightly further away from work or getting off the bus a stop early. Aim to build up to a moderate level of activity – moderate means you will feel slightly out of breath but are still able to hold a conversation. And remember to warm up and cool down properly to reduce risk of injury.

Do something you enjoy

If the idea of going to the gym fills you with dread, signing up to an expensive membership you know you won't use probably isn't the best idea. I do ashtanga yoga because I enjoy it, I can do it in the comfort of my own home, it fits around my family and work life and I enjoy the sense of balance it brings to my life. But if you

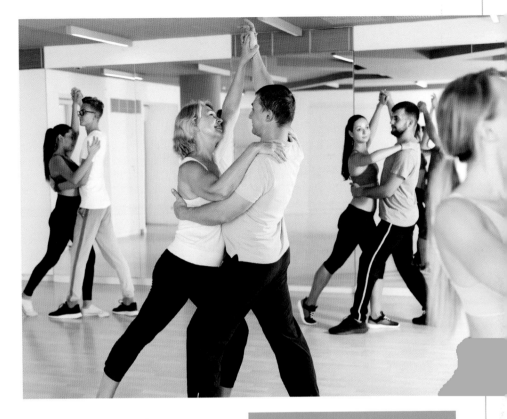

↑ Finding an activity you enjoy is the key to success.

told me I'd have to do step aerobics or go running then I'd tell you to forget it! It's so important to find something you enjoy and then you'll be more likely to stick to it.

Buddy up

If your willpower is waning, try exercising with a friend to boost motivation and burn calories. A University of Aberdeen study found that exercising with a companion increased the amount of exercise people took. This was boosted further when the exercise buddy was emotionally supportive.[48]

Menopause-friendly diet

Diet can be overlooked during your perimenopause and menopause. Tiredness or low mood could leave you reaching for a sugary treat to get through the day. Or your favourite spicy foods or evening glass of wine might trigger hot flushes, meaning that you don't get the same enjoyment from food you once did. Yet eating a balanced diet is as important as ever.

If you are unsure what a balanced diet should look like, a good starting point is a Mediterranean-style diet featuring plenty of fruit, vegetables and wholegrains like rice and pasta. A Mediterranean diet includes fish and poultry, is low in red meat and processed foods and favours unsaturated fats found in olive oil and nuts.

How will healthy eating help me through my menopause?

Eating a balanced diet has a multitude of benefits, enabling you to:

- protect your bones: with both calcium and vitamin D key for maintaining and strengthening your bones
- maintain a healthy weight: studies have shown that being obese can increase menopausal symptoms such as hot flushes and joint and muscular pain[18]
- boost your mood and energy levels without resorting to sugary snacks.

How much do I need?

Government guidelines say women need 700mg of calcium a day, which you should be able to get from your diet.[49]

Why calcium is key

As our bone density reduces during the perimenopause and menopause, its essential to eat a diet with plenty of the mineral calcium to keep our bones strong and healthy. Calcium-rich foods include:

- milk, cheese and yoghurt (including low-fat versions)
- green, leafy vegetables
- bony fish, such as sardines, pilchards and tinned salmon
- nuts
- tofu
- soya beans
- breakfast cereals and non-dairy milks fortified with calcium.

The sunshine vitamin

Vitamin D helps our bodies absorb calcium, so in turn keeps our bones strong. You should get all the vitamin D you need from sunlight on your skin, your diet and supplements, if needed.

In the UK, most of your vitamin D will come from direct sunlight exposure from late March or early April to September. How much time you need in the sun to make enough vitamin D varies from person to person. You should be able to get enough from short sun exposure while going about your daily life, but never let your skin redden or burn.[50]

Foods containing vitamin D include:

- oily fish like salmon, mackerel and sardines
- red meat
- eggs
- cereals and fortified foods.

It is hard to get your daily vitamin D requirement from food alone, so current government advice is that all adults (and children) should take a daily vitamin D supplement, particularly during autumn and winter. If you are at a higher risk of vitamin D deficiency (if, for example, you don't go outdoors much or your clothes cover most of your skin when outside) then you should consider taking a supplement all year round. If you are from an African, African-Caribbean or South Asian background then you should also consider a year-round supplement.[49]

Reduce your sugar intake

It is easy to reach for a quick sugar boost when you are tired or feeling low. But menopause or no menopause, we could all benefit from reducing sugar in our diet. A 2018 study found that adults in England are eating double the recommended amount of the sweet stuff.[52]

Government guidelines say that no more than 5% of the energy (or calories) you get from food should be made up of 'free sugars'.[52] Free sugars are the sugars

added to food by manufacturers and sugars naturally present in honey, syrups and fruit juice (sugars naturally found in milk, fruit and vegetables are not included).[53] For women, this equates to no more than 30g – or seven teaspoons – of free sugars a day.

If you are relying on sugar to give you an energy boost, try eating wholegrain foods such as brown rice and oats. Wholegrain foods are high in fibre, help to keep you fuller for longer and release energy more slowly than sugary foods.

⬇ Omega 3 in fish provides numerous health benefits including lowering future risk of heart diease.

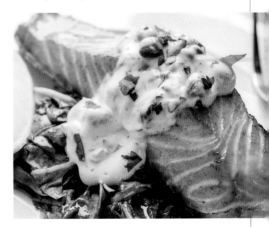

> ## Did you know?
>
> *Government guidelines say that adults should consume no more than 30g – seven teaspoons – of free sugars a day.*

Do I need to take supplements?

There is no substitute for a healthy, varied diet, but some women may benefit from the following supplements.

Magnesium

Magnesium is a very important mineral, which is actually responsible for over 300 enzyme reactions and is found in all of our tissues, especially in our bones, muscles and brain. Our cells need magnesium to make energy, for many different chemical pumps to work, to stabilise membranes and also to help muscles relax.

Many people have magnesium

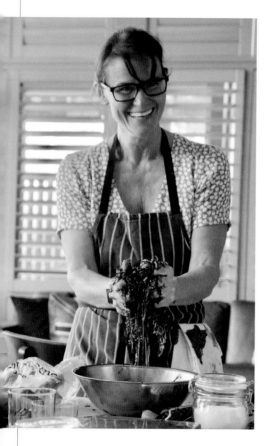

deficiency, as they are eating diets that contain practically no magnesium. Processed foods, meat and dairy food contain very little or no magnesium. Drinking alcohol and coffee, certain medications, such as water tablets and antibiotics, and also stress can all reduce magnesium absorption.

You should get most of the magnesium you need from your diet, including green leafy vegetables, brown rice and wholegrains. Nuts such as almonds, cashews and peanuts are packed with magnesium and are a healthy snack.

There are different types of magnesium available as supplements. The most absorbable forms are magnesium citrate, glycinate taurate or aspartate. Other beneficial types are magnesium malate, succinate and fumarate. Taking a magnesium supplement with vitamin B can improve its absorption. Government guidelines say women 19–64 years need 270mg a day.[49]

Many people find that taking a good quality magnesium supplement can improve sleep and lower stress levels. Magnesium is linked to greater bone density in women. It can also improve sleep and headaches, reduce anxiety and can also help soothe muscular and joint pains.

← Emma Ellice-Flint provides nutritional therapy at my menopause and wellbeing centre

Omega 3

Omega 3 polyunsaturated fatty acids have a wide range of health benefits. There is increasing research which demonstrates that taking omega 3 can reduce vasomotor menopausal symptoms and heart disease, without increasing risk of cancer. Oily fish like mackerel and kippers are a main source of omega 3 (as well as linseeds and omega 3-enriched eggs) but if you don't eat fish then you may want to consider a supplement.

Look after your gut

We are what we eat, as the old adage goes. And it may surprise you that there is a link between a healthy gut and hormone health. Hormone receptors in the gut help with the function of the bowel, and during your perimenopause and menopause, you may suffer from bloating or poor digestion due to hormone imbalances affecting the balance of bacteria in your gut.

Eating a balanced diet with plenty of fibre encourages the growth of 'good' bacteria, which not only play a role in our digestion but also in our energy levels, immunity and weight. Good bacteria are also linked to levels of the brain chemical serotonin, which can improve mood.

What foods are good for my gut?

Foods that are good for gut health can be divided into two broad types:

1 Prebiotics – foods that stimulate the growth of good bacteria in your gut.

2 Probiotics – live bacteria and yeasts thought to help restore the natural balance of bacteria in your gut when it has been disrupted by an illness or treatment.[54]

Emma Ellice-Flint BHSc is a clinical nutritionist and former chef who provides nutritional therapy at my centre. While it is always best to consult a professional in case of any of food intolerances, Emma recommends the following:

◆ Prebiotic foods, which can include: garlic, onions, asparagus, chicory, radicchio, artichoke, cocoa, ginger, cabbage, fennel, beetroot, bananas, blueberries, apples.

◆ Probiotic foods, which can include: kefir, live yoghurt, kombucha, sauerkraut, kimchi, natto and live apple cider vinegar.

Probiotic supplements can also help correct the imbalance of bacteria in the gut and I often advise looking for a probiotic that is easily absorbed with a high bacteria count. *Lactobacillus acidophilus* is a probiotic bacteria normally found in your intestines and crucial to health. Because of its ability to produce lactic acid and to interact with your immune system, it may help prevent and treat symptoms of various diseases including irritable bowel syndrome, some allergies, and may even help to reduce cholesterol levels.

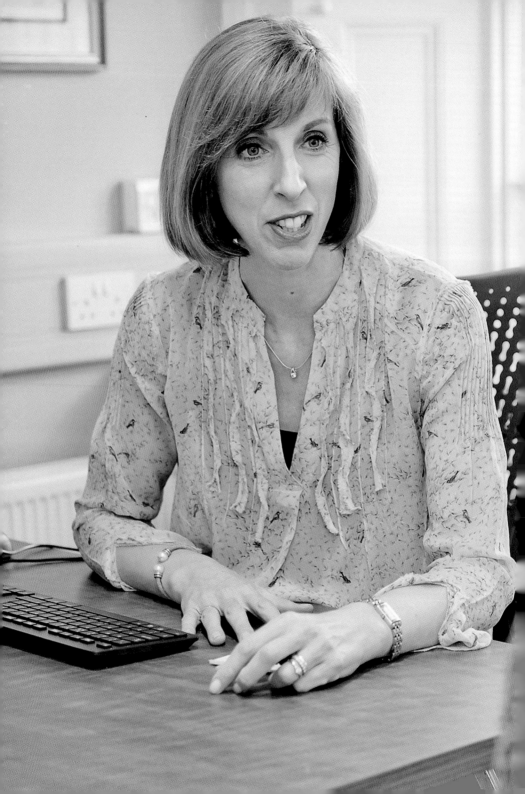

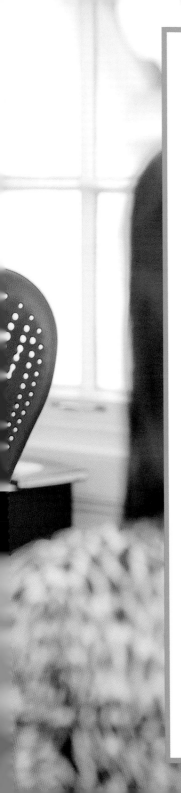

Chapter 5

Get the most out of your appointment

Countless women have sat and sobbed in despair in my clinic. However, many women have returned a few months later and wept with relief and joy that they feel well again. Making an appointment to see a health professional about troublesome symptoms is often a crucial step in getting your life back. It's a chance to get a diagnosis and have a discussion with a professional (usually your GP) so you can make an informed decision on the right treatment for you.

This should be a positive experience and should herald the beginning of some blessed relief from your symptoms. Yet some women face months or even years of additional suffering because of an uphill battle in accessing correct information and treatment. This is because their GP doesn't have a true understanding of treatments like HRT and how they can help, and this has to change. One campaign calling for such changes is #MakeMenopauseMatter, spearheaded by Menopause Support's Diane Danzebrink, who has campaigned tirelessly for greater awareness.

The #MakeMenopauseMatter campaign has three key aims; to improve menopause training amongst GPs, to raise awareness of menopause in the workplace (including all employers to having menopause guidelines to support women), and to introduce menopause education into the curriculum for teenagers.

This chapter will help empower you to get the right information and treatment for your symptoms, including:

- ◆ When and where to get help
- ◆ Preparing for your first appointment
- ◆ Overcoming obstacles, and what to do if your doctor won't listen.

When you need to see a doctor

So far we have covered the causes, signs and symptoms of the perimenopause and menopause. And we know about the treatments and lifestyle changes that can make a real difference.

Not every woman will have a difficult menopause. But if you suspect you are perimenopausal or menopausal and find that symptoms are getting in the way of everyday life, now is the time to see your doctor or a healthcare professional with a special interest in the menopause.

A 2016 British Menopause Society study revealed that one in two British women aged 45–65 with menopausal symptoms had gone through their menopause without consulting a healthcare professional about their symptoms.[55] This was despite the women surveyed reporting on average seven different symptoms and 42% admitting they were worse or much worse than expected.

Please don't suffer in silence or resort to self-managing troublesome symptoms. Ring and make an appointment today.

Who should I see?

In most cases, your first port of call will be your local surgery, where you can speak to a doctor or practice nurse about your symptoms and treatment options. It is worth asking if there is a person who specialises in the menopause in your surgery.

If you have a complex medical history, or POI is suspected, or if treatment doesn't seem to be working, then you may be referred to a specialist menopause clinic. A menopause clinic is usually made up of doctors, nurses and counsellors trained in menopause management. Another option is to go to a private menopause clinic like mine. The majority of women who I see self-refer, so they do not need a referral from another doctor.

The British Menopause Society has a UK-wide register of recognised menopause specialists, covering people working in both NHS and private clinics and services. A menopause specialist is a healthcare professional who, like myself, is a member of the Society and has specialist competency in menopause. There are just over 40 NHS or private menopause clinics in the UK. To find your nearest one, go to the Society's website (https://thebms.org.uk/find-a-menopause-specialist).

Preparing for your appointment

Medical appointments can be frustratingly short, with a 2017 study revealing that average UK GP appointments are among the shortest in Europe at just 9.2 minutes.[56] There is nothing worse than feeling rushed or being unable to communicate your concerns. After working as a GP for 18 years, I know how difficult it is to assess someone's needs when you are limited to a ten-minute consultation. The following pages contain tips to help you get the best out of your appointment.

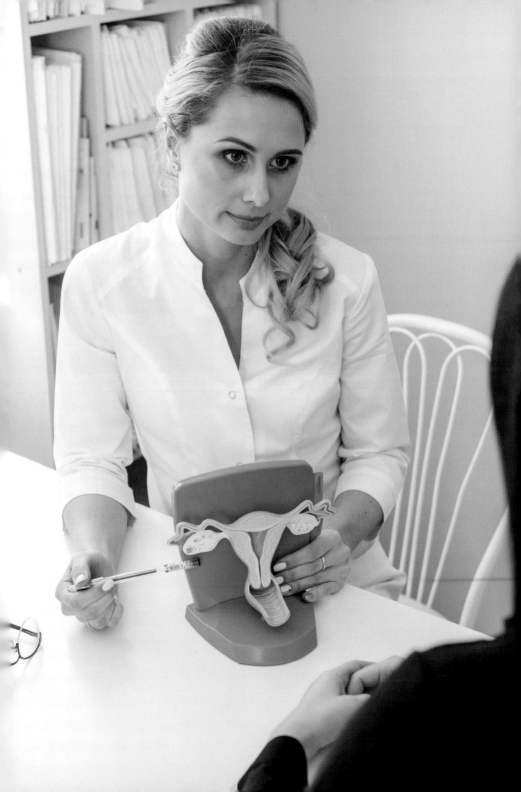

What should happen at my appointment?

The 2015 NICE menopause guidelines state that your GP should discuss with you (and family members if appropriate):

- the stages of menopause
- common symptoms and how the menopause is diagnosed
- lifestyle changes that could help your health and wellbeing
- benefits and risks of treatments for menopausal symptoms (this includes HRT, non-hormonal treatments such as clonidine and other treatments like CBT)
- how the menopause may affect your future health.[26]

What about follow-ups?

NICE guidelines recommend a review three months after your initial appointment. Provided that you don't have any issues, you can then move to annual reviews, but ask for a review earlier if you are experiencing side effects of any treatments, or if your treatment doesn't seem to be working.

At the end of the appointment

Try to leave the consulting room with as many questions answered as possible. What is the next stage? When will you need to come back? Who do you contact with further questions?

Ask for take-home material such as leaflets. Make a note of what was discussed and note any follow-up appointments in your diary.

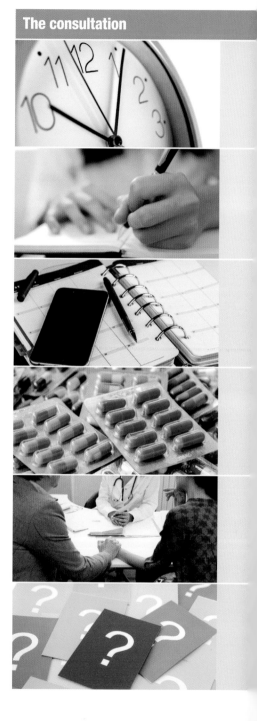

The consultation

Ask for a double appointment

Some surgeries offer this option for more complex appointments that will take more than 10 minutes. These appointments may be in short supply, so try to book well in advance. Often, surgeries will have a doctor or practice nurse who is interested in the menopause and women's health, so ask to see them when making an appointment.

Write down your symptoms

At my clinic, we ask women to fill out a questionnaire called the Greene Climacteric Scale,[57] which you can see in Appendix 1 of this manual. This is a standard checklist used by many health professionals worldwide to record menopausal symptoms women may be experiencing. Fill out the checklist before your own appointment for an at-a-glance list of the nature and severity of your symptoms. It will help to pinpoint your more troublesome symptoms so you can talk about these first.

Bring your diary

Your health professional should be able to tell if you are in your perimenopause or menopause based on your age, symptoms and how often you have periods. Remember that FSH blood testing can be unreliable, so you are unlikely to need tests unless you are under 45 years of age. Specifics help. Keep a note of key changes such as period frequency and flow, sleep quality and duration and bring to your appointment.

Have a list of any medication you are taking

This should include prescription medication and any herbal medicines or supplements.

Feeling nervous? Take a friend

Moral support can really help to reduce anxiety. Brief your friend beforehand on the most important things you want to get across in your appointment so they can prompt you if you forget.

Don't be afraid to ask questions

If you don't understand something or aren't getting the information you want, speak up. NICE has compiled a list of suggested questions, such as 'Are there any treatments suitable for my symptoms?' and 'Are there any support organisations in my local area?'[58]

Overcoming obstacles

I've started treatment but it isn't working: what now?

Treatments such as HRT, vaginal estrogen, testosterone and non-hormonal treatments like vaginal moisturisers generally can take a few months to work. However, if you feel like your symptoms aren't improving, or you are experiencing unwanted side effects, go back. It might be that the dose or type of treatment needs to be adjusted (this is quite common in the first few months of HRT) or you need to try a different treatment altogether.

If treatments just aren't working, you are entitled to ask for a second opinion. You could ask about a referral to a specialist health professional with an interest in menopause. Specialist menopause clinics do fantastic work, but unfortunately there just aren't enough of them to meet demand and waiting times can be long.

My GP will only offer me antidepressants, but I'm not depressed

Sadly, women often tell me this is the case. The NICE guidelines are clear that antidepressants are not effective for menopause-related mood changes, so point this out and ask why they want you to take antidepressants. Take along the NICE guidance to refer to.

Note: certain types of antidepressants such as citalopram or venlafaxine may be offered if you have hot flushes and are unable or don't want to take HRT.

> ### Did you know?
>
> *One in two women with menopausal symptoms don't see a health professional.*[55]

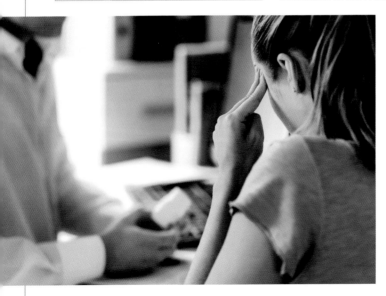

← If your symptoms aren't improving or you are experiencing side effects, make a follow up appointment.

→ Remember you are entitled to ask for a second opinion.

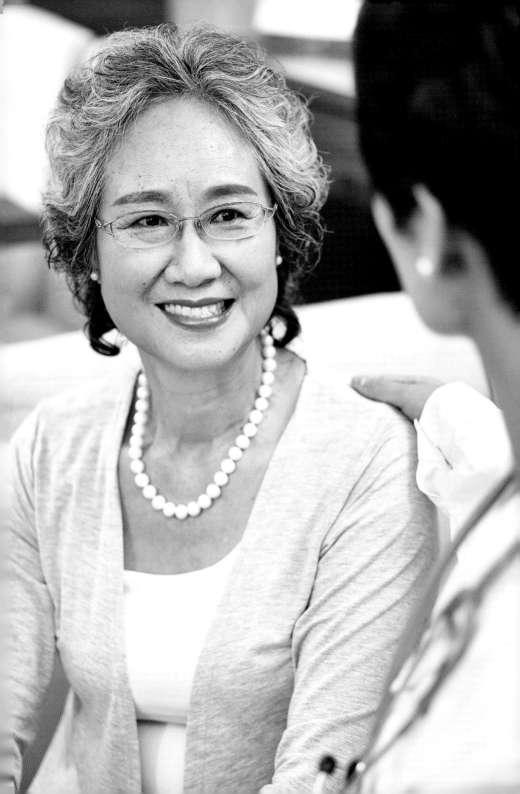

I want to take HRT, but my doctor refuses to prescribe it: what can I do?

I'm not going to claim that HRT is a panacea for every woman's every menopausal symptom. Some women don't want to take it and others can't for medical reasons. But for those willing and able, HRT shouldn't be dismissed out of hand. The NICE guidelines are clear: for most women, the benefits of HRT outweigh the risks. But the initial findings of the Women's Health Initiative study persist to this day, even though numerous studies published since have debunked so many of the issues it appeared to raise.

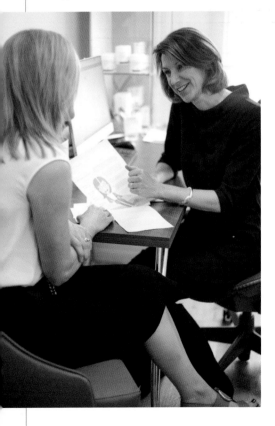

Many doctors and healthcare professionals continue to be fixated by the idea that HRT, cancer, blood clots and heart problems go hand in hand, which is clearly incorrect. We have many patients who travel long distances to my clinic in Stratford-upon-Avon because their GPs won't prescribe HRT.

Many doctors are still depriving women of medication that would have cost the NHS just £4 a month, and that has the ability to give women their lives back and improve their future health. This should not be happening now that we have menopause guidelines.

Many patients tell us in the clinic that their doctors have cited outdated scare stories of an increased risk of breast cancer, or that antidepressants would probably help, or that they would have to 'brave it out' as the menopause is just a natural process. This is exactly the sort of mindset that we all need to challenge. You may feel like you are being a nuisance, but if there is no medical reason why HRT is unsuitable for you, then it is essential to speak up.

Healthcare professionals are compassionate people with your best interests at heart, and they should be willing to listen to your reasoning and answer your questions. If a face-to-face discussion outlining your concerns doesn't work, then it may help to put things down in writing.

Get a second opinion

You could ask to speak to another health professional at the same surgery or ask for a referral to a specialist. You are entitled to have a second opinion from a different doctor. Another option is self-referring to a private menopause clinic.

Example letter to GP requesting HRT

Here is a sample letter from my website that women have used to good success. One lady who works in West Midlands Police had tried four different antidepressants and then after five years realised her symptoms were related to her menopause. She was repeatedly refused HRT and then took in this letter. She has now taken HRT for six months and feels so much better; and she has been promoted at work too.

(insert your name and address)
(insert date)

Dear Dr (name)

Please don't think I am trying to tell you your job because I am not. I really respect you; you listen, you are very thorough, you have excellent people skills and you always show compassion and empathy. I am writing as I would really like to take HRT.

I feel I have a good knowledge of the menopause as I have read information on the Menopause Support website (www.menopausesupport.co.uk) and that of their medical adviser Dr Louise Newson, a GP who specialises in the menopause (www.menopausedoctor.co.uk). I have also read through the NICE guidance on menopause.

Can I ask if the reason for not supporting this treatment is a financial one or for health reasons?

I would really appreciate it if the practice would consider me having HRT as I know the benefits of HRT are more likely to outweigh any risks for me.

Please can you contact me when you have read this letter and looked at the NICE guidelines to let me know if there is any other way you can support me? If there is no other option available via my GP, then I may have to look at what other options are available to me so I can try and address the symptoms I am experiencing and move forward.

Many thanks for taking the time to read this letter; I look forward to hearing from you in due course.

Yours sincerely,

(insert your name and sign above it)
(insert your date of birth)

Why we need to get things right

All women deserve access to good menopause advice and care. I've met and worked alongside numerous expert doctors, nurses, pharmacists, therapists and administrative staff who are dedicated to improving the health and wellbeing of women.

So it both astonishes and dismays me when I hear from so many women that they are being denied treatments without a valid medical reason, or are being wrongly prescribed treatments like antidepressants for their mood symptoms. This often leads to them resorting to self-managing their symptoms, and it is not uncommon for them to spend huge amounts of money on ineffective or potentially dangerous medications.

This is not good enough and it has to change. And that starts with better menopause education across the board – for doctors, nurses, pharmacists and also for women. I have lectured at the Royal College of General Practitioners, I provide e-learning sessions for doctors, and we hold medical education events at my clinic. It is great to be able to bring their understanding of HRT up to date, because so many of them qualified in an era when HRT was demonised and, as a result, they still don't have the confidence to prescribe it.

There is a real thirst for knowledge among doctors and nurses and this needs to be matched with good, evidence-based menopause education at undergraduate level. Every woman who walks through the door of a surgery, clinic or ward will go through the menopause one day. An investment in better menopause education at undergraduate and postgraduate levels is an investment in the future health of all women.

For more information

British Menopause Society:
www.thebms.org.uk

Daisy Network:
www.daisynetwork.org

Faculty of Sexual and Reproductive:
Health: www.fsrh.org

International Menopause Society:
www.imsociety.org

My Menopause Doctor:
www.menopausedoctor.co.uk

NICE menopause guidelines:
www.nice.org.uk/guidance/ng23

Primary Care Women's Health Forum:
www.pcwhf.co.uk

Royal College of Nursing:
www.rcn.org.uk

Royal College of Obstetricians and
Gynaecologists: www.rcog.org.uk

Why all health professionals need to be menopause aware

All women deserve access to good menopause care and advice. Without it, women are in danger of not getting the treatment they need.

I have met and worked alongside numerous expert doctors, nurses, pharmacists, therapists and administrative staff who are dedicated to improving the health and wellbeing of perimenopausal and menopausal women.

However there still remains a real need for improved menopause education across the board for healthcare professionals.

There is a thirst for knowledge and this needs to be matched with good, evidence-based education at undergraduate and also at a postgraduate level. After all, every woman who walks through the door of a surgery, clinic or pharmacy will go through her menopause one day.

My not for profit organisation, Newson Health Research and Education, has worked with FourteenFish (fourteenfish.com) and developed a menopause education programme for health professionals, especially those working in primary care.

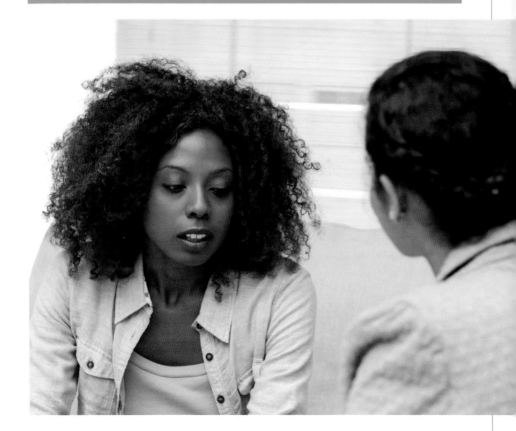

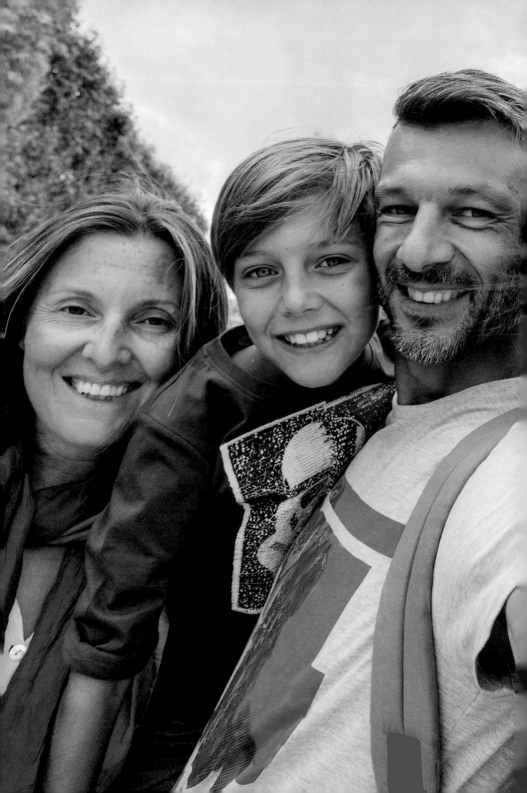

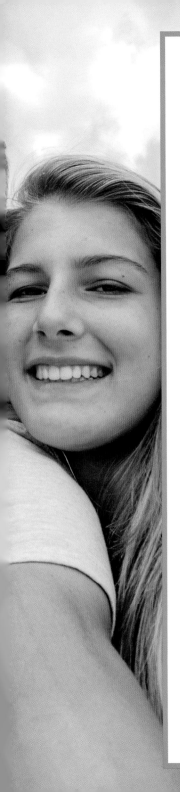

Chapter 6

Relationships and your menopause

Your menopause can be an isolating time and it can feel like no one understands what you are going through. The temptation is to hide away and wait for it all to be over, but shutting loved ones out is the worst thing you can do. Being open and honest during this time could actually help to strengthen your bond with your partner, children and friends – and help you to realise that you are not alone. We have also included some tips for your loved ones in Appendix 2.

In this chapter we will be looking at how to menopause-proof your relationships, including:

◆ Educating your family and friends
◆ Clash of the hormones: menopause and teenage children
◆ Sex and your menopause.

Don't go it alone

Even the closest bonds of family and friendship can be tested to their limits during your menopause.

Hormones can wreak havoc with our moods and can leave us angry one minute and tearful the next. And when you add physical symptoms to the mix, it is perhaps no surprise that I have treated numerous women whose relationships have either failed or are failing as a result of their menopause. I have no doubt the menopause plays a part in high divorce rates of couples in their mid to late 40s.

Women tell me how their relationships have been put under strain due to their symptoms, and they find themselves lashing out or becoming cross for no reason. One woman told me she had

such uncontrollable rage at times that, had she had a knife in her hand, she would have stabbed her husband.

Many women say friendships suffer as they have no energy or motivation for seeing even their closest girlfriends. And mothers tell me how they have no patience with their offspring – particularly those with teenagers. Raising a teenager can be challenging at the best of times, not least of all when you are going through your menopause.

As the mother of three daughters, I know how it feels. Before the penny dropped that I was perimenopausal, I was becoming increasingly short-tempered with my

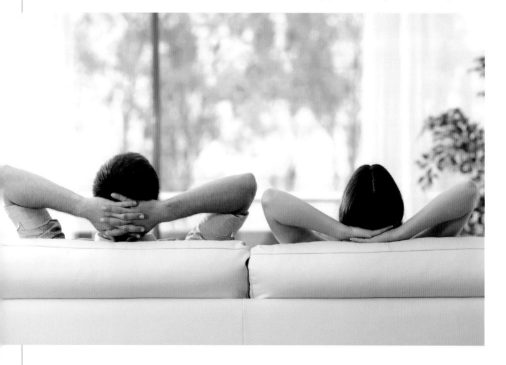

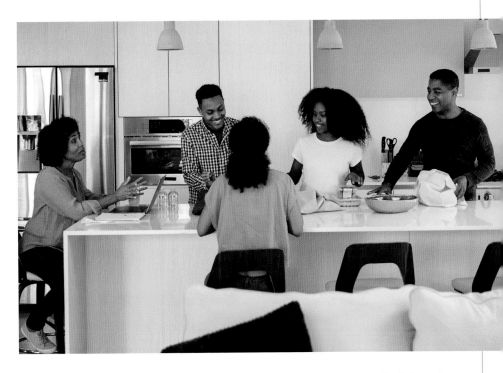

husband and children. I was constantly shouting at my husband over trivial matters, even though in hindsight he had done nothing wrong. There were times I felt so irritable that even the sound of my husband's breathing annoyed me!

Those closest to us can also feel confused and often helpless, so it is vital that you keep communication channels open. Although it may be hard to see the positives from your menopause when you are struggling with symptoms, remember – this period of your life is finite. We spend an average of one-third of our lives postmenopausal, so see this time as an opportunity to improve your relationships.

Explore treatment options

Don't underestimate the positive effect the right treatment could have on your symptoms. If you haven't already, go to see a health professional and talk through options available to you so you can make an informed choice.

Education, education, education

Much of the information available about menopause is outdated or inaccurate, so it is often down to us to educate our loved ones. I'm not proposing that you call long-lost relatives in Australia to tell them about your hot flushes or moods, but it is really important to be frank with close friends and family. Signpost credible sources of information (such as this manual, my menopausedoctor.co.uk website, the NHS Choices website and NICE guidelines) and ask if they have any questions.

Your menopause is a normal, natural event, and we all need to normalise it by talking about it. Tell people about your

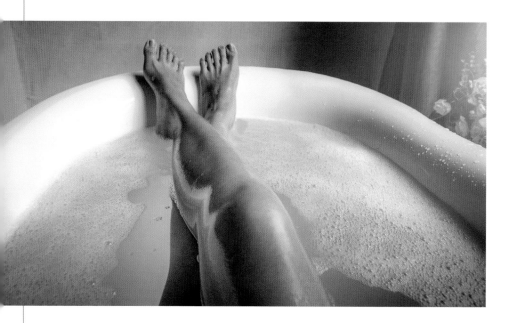

symptoms and how they can best support you. What is it that you need? A listening ear, or more practical help such as taking on tasks that you don't have the headspace for?

Be honest

Talking is the single most effective way you can help those around you to understand your menopause. Try to put things into perspective for them. If you are feeling overwhelmed when you walk through the door in the evening, or quick to irritate during a catch-up with friends, say why. 'I'm feeling terrible today because I've had no sleep/my joints ache/I'm having a hot flush' is better than family and friends feeling bewildered or trying to second guess what is wrong.

Don't be afraid to say no

Sometimes the best way to relax will be surrounding yourself with loved ones and laughter. Yet there may be times that you

just can't face that social occasion in a hot, crowded bar, or having your extended family over for Sunday lunch is the final straw. If you don't want to, say no. Your friends will understand and your family can cope without you for one day.

Seize the opportunity to take time for yourself – take a long bath, read a book, exercise, phone a friend. Whatever it is that makes you happy and leaves you refreshed.

My relationship isn't working: what now?

The divorce rate is highest among couples aged 45–49 in England and Wales,[60] and I have no doubt that the strain the menopause can put on relationships plays a part. A lot of women find that relationship counselling can help. The charity Relate offers relationship counselling for individuals and couples, and also has some useful resources on its website about general relationship issues, sex and the menopause (www.relate.org.uk).

Be a menopause friend

These days, there is a whole industry dedicated to all things pregnancy and parenting, including websites, apps and meet up groups. We need just as much support during our menopause years. Talking things over with those who are going through the same thing can be a real source of comfort.

Many women tell me that while they are comfortable talking about periods, pregnancy and parenting, the menopause remains an off-limits topic among friends. It is likely that others in your own circle of friends are facing the perimenopause or menopause just like you. Be the one to break the taboo. Next time you have an outing with your friends, bring up your menopause. Find out if others are going through the same thing and suggest being each other's support network.

Try setting up a WhatsApp group to swap stories and coping strategies. Sending a quick message can be a good way to vent, ask advice and offer words of encouragement to others in the group. Some friends might not want to talk or haven't yet reached this stage. But just knowing there's support there if and when they do want to talk will be a comfort.

You could also look outside your friendship group for ways of boosting your support network. I am a medical adviser for the Latte Lounge, a virtual coffee shop where women over 40 discuss issues such as health and relationships. There's lots of discussion about menopause on the Latte Lounge's Facebook groups and menopause information on the main website (www.lattelounge.co).

You could also try Menopause Café, a non-for-profit network of discussion groups where women and men share stories and ask questions about the menopause over a cup of tea (menopausecafe.net).

Menopause Support is a great website set up by Diane Danzebrink, a therapist, coach and menopause expert with nurse training in menopause. She also holds workshops for women covering all things menopause (www.menopausesupport.co.uk).

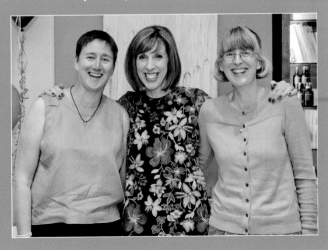

➜ From left: Diane Danzebrink, Dr Louise Newson and author and menopause campaigner Jane Lewis.

Let's talk about sex: menopause and your love life

Of all menopausal symptoms, low libido is one women often feel embarrassed to talk about, even those who I have known for many years.

One woman recently told me how she felt like her libido had 'vanished … as though someone had switched a light off'. If your libido has taken a nosedive, you are not alone. A survey of 2,500 peri- and postmenopausal women found that 84% thought that having an active sex life was important, but 79% said the menopause transition affected their libido. Of those who had a lower sex drive, just 27% had discussed this issue with health professionals.[61]

My advice? Don't be embarrassed about talking to a heath professional. I know it is a sensitive issue, but we are there to help you, not pass judgement on your sex life (or lack thereof).

Find a treatment to suit you

HRT can typically help restore your libido within a couple of months. Do be mindful that taking estrogen as a tablet can increase levels of sex hormone binding globulin. This binds to testosterone and, as a result can lower libido, but this doesn't happen if you use estrogen patches, gels or sprays. You could also talk to your health professional about testosterone if you are taking HRT and you feel it is not helping your libido.

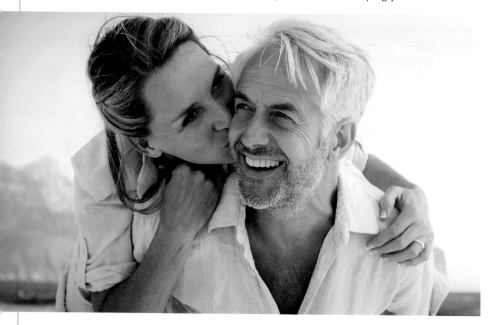

Testosterone is usually given as a cream or gel and can be taken alongside HRT, and you should notice improvements within a couple of months.

Get moving

Exercise releases endorphins: feel-good chemicals that improve our mood. Exercise also increases blood flow to the vagina, which in turn improves sensitivity. A study of 370 Brazilian women aged 40–65 found that those who were physically active reported higher levels of desire, arousal, lubrication, orgasm and satisfaction than women who were only moderately active or sedentary.[62]

The power of touch and the 'love hormone'

There's more to intimacy than just sex. Hugging releases oxytocin, a soothing hormone nicknamed the 'love hormone', which promotes recognition, trust and sexual arousal.[63] Kissing, hugging or just holding hands are all ways to maintain physical contact.

If you find sex painful, foreplay will increase natural lubrication, or you may find that a lubricant also helps. You could try experimenting with different positions to find what is comfortable for you, or invest in some sex toys. Jo Divine is an online sex toy company founded by trained nurse Samantha Evans (www.jodivine.com). The site includes lots of advice and product suggestions for menopausal women.

Make time for two

Juggling a career, and perhaps children and caring responsibilities for older parents, may mean there is little time for romance in your lives. If your home is less love nest, more house of chaos, why not try escaping for a night in a hotel?

Look after your pelvic floor

Pelvic floor exercises can help with bladder weakness, and research shows it can intensify orgasms (see Chapter 2).

How to beat vaginal dryness

Not only does it cause you physical discomfort, but vaginal atrophy and the related symptoms of dryness, irritation and inflammation can be a real barrier to a healthy sex life (see Chapter 2). A study presented at the North American Menopause Society annual meeting in 2017 looked at the impact vaginal atrophy and bladder problems had on women's sex lives. The questionnaire of 1,500 women revealed that fear of experiencing pain during sex was reported as a reason for restricting or avoiding sex altogether, more than a fear of having to interrupt sex to go to the toilet.[64]

Vaginal dryness is one of the symptoms that can persist after your menopause has ended. But the good news is there are a whole host of treatments – both hormonal and non-hormonal – that you can try to help keep these symptoms at bay.

Topical estrogen is available on

Did you know?

You can also help to prevent vaginal dryness by avoiding heavily perfumed products or washing powders that can cause irritation.

Treatments for vaginal dryness

Treatment	Contains hormones?	How is it used?	How often is it used?	Prescription only?
HRT	Yes	Tablet, patch, gel or spray	Depends on the type and dosage	Yes
Estrogen cream	Yes	Cream applied to affected area	Every day for first 2 weeks, twice weekly thereafter	Yes
Estrogen vaginal tablet	Yes	Very small tablet inserted with applicator	Every day for first 2 weeks, usually twice weekly thereafter	Yes
Estrogen ring	Yes	Soft, flexible ring is inserted by you, doctor or nurse. Releases steady, low dose of estrogen	Should be replaced every 3 months	Yes
Vaginal moisturiser	No	Applied to vagina using either prefilled or reusable applicators	Varies between brands but usually once every three days	No
Water-based and oil-based lubricants	No	Applied before sex. Water-based products are compatible with natural rubber and latex condoms and toys	As and when needed	No

prescription. Remember, using topical tablet, cream or a ring delivers estrogen directly to the vagina so is not the same as taking HRT and does not have the same associated risks. It can be safely used for long periods of time, which is reassuring as you may find your symptoms return if you stop this treatment. You could also try vaginal moisturisers, non-hormone creams that keep the tissues hydrated, and a lubricant during sex to relieve discomfort. The best makes are YES, Sylk and Regelle. Some of the other types can actually cause more irritation and discomfort. These can be bought over the counter or online.

Contraception Q&A

Our fertility naturally decreases with age and, although getting pregnant is less likely during your perimenopause and menopause, it is still possible. You can still ovulate (produce an egg) when you are having periods, even when they are irregular, so contraception is important to avoid unwanted pregnancy. Getting pregnant over 40 increases your risk of complications such as miscarriage, gestational diabetes, high blood pressure and chromosomal conditions such as Down's syndrome.[59]

How long do I need to take contraception for?

According to current guidelines from the Faculty of Sexual and Reproductive Healthcare (FSRH),[59] if you are:

- under 50, you should use contraception for at least two years following your last menstrual period
- over 50, use contraception for at least one year following your last menstrual period.

All women can stop contraception at 55, as getting pregnant after this age is exceptionally rare, even in women still having periods.

What is the best type of contraception for me?

What is best for you depends on your age, lifestyle factors and any pre-existing medication conditions and should be discussed with a health professional.

- **The combined pill** contains estrogen and progestogen. As well as providing protection against pregnancy, it can help to regulate periods, tackle period pains and ease menopausal symptoms such as hot flushes and night sweats and maintain bone density.[65] FSRH guidelines say it can be taken up until the age of 50,[59] but is not suitable:
  - ◇ if you are aged over 35 years and a smoker
  - ◇ are aged 40 or over and have cardiovascular disease or a history of blood clots, stroke or migraine.

If contraception is still needed after you reach 50, then you should switch to a

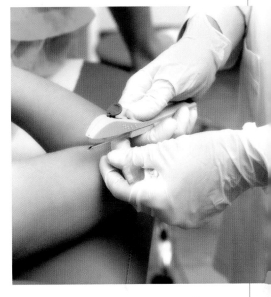

↑ The implant is a type of contraceptive placed under the skin in your upper arm and lasts for three years.

safer, alternative method such as the progestogen-only pill.

- **The progestogen-only pill** has fewer risks associated with it and can usually be taken up to the age of 55. It also makes periods lighter and can stop them altogether.
- **The implant** is a small plastic rod placed under your skin in your upper arm. It releases progestogen into the bloodstream and works for three years. The progestogen-only implant and the progestogen-only pill are not associated with increased risks of clot, stroke or heart attack. The implant can be used until the age of 50.
- **The injection** releases progestogen into the bloodstream and is usually administered every three months. It can be used until the age of 50.

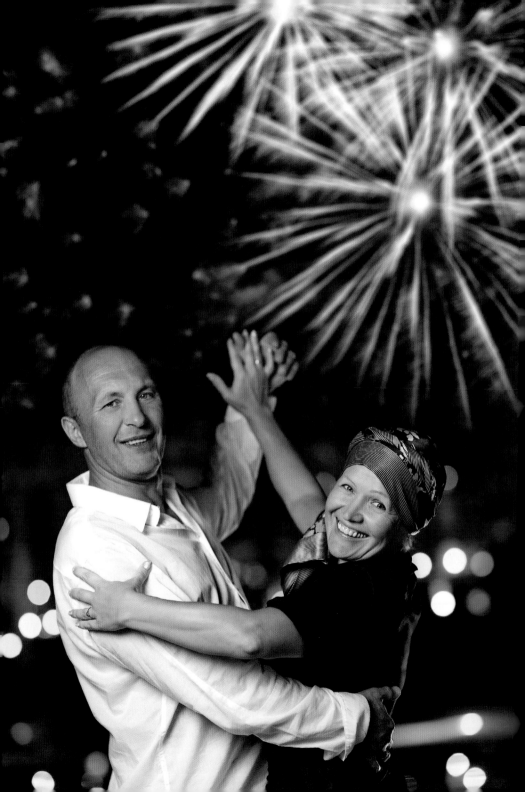

- **The intrauterine contraceptive device (IUCD or ICD)**, more commonly known as the coil, is made from copper and is hormone free. It is inserted into your uterus by a doctor or nurse and works by making it more difficult for sperm to reach an egg, or stopping a fertilised egg implanting in the uterus. Although it is hormone free, it can make periods heavier.
- **The intrauterine system (IUS)** is a plastic coil containing a progestogen, which is inserted into your uterus in a similar way to an IUCD. It releases a progestogen at a slow but constant rate and thins the lining of your uterus, so it is less likely to accept a fertilised egg.[67] The IUS (Mirena is the brand usually used in the UK) can be also used as the progestogen element of HRT. If it is used in this way, it should be changed every five years. If it is used for contraception only, the IUS can be used up until the age of 55 (if fitted when you are aged 45 or over).

I'm taking contraception: how will I know when my periods have stopped?

While taking contraception doesn't delay or alter the duration of your menopause, it can mask the signs and symptoms. If you are using a progestogen-only contraception, a side effect can be reduced or no bleeding at all, so it can be difficult to know when your menopause occurs. If you are taking the combined contraceptive pill, then your 'periods' are actually withdrawal bleeds related to hormones rather than your own menstrual cycle.

If you are uncertain when your last period was, you can ask for a blood test to be taken to check your FSH levels. If the level of this hormone is elevated, then you will need to continue using contraception for two years if you are under 50 years old and one year if you are over 50 years old.

If you are using the IUS or progestogen-only pill, there is no need to remove or stop these prior to testing, but if you are on the combined contraceptive pill you will need to stop taking it at least six weeks before the test to get an accurate result.

High doses of progestogens, such as those seen in the injection, may affect the FSH result, so please discuss this with your health professional.

Can HRT be used for contraception?

As HRT contains very low levels of hormones, it does not work as a contraceptive. If you are taking HRT then you can also take the progesterone-only pill or have an IUCD or IUS inserted if you require contraception. However, if you are taking a type of HRT that does not lead to periods then contraception is usually not necessary.

Don't forget about sexually transmitted infections

A UK survey found that 8.9% of women aged 45–54 and 4.4% of women aged 55–64 had at least one new sexual partner in the previous year.[59] Even if you are taking contraception, remember that condoms are the only way to protect against sexually transmitted infections.

When hormones collide: your menopause & teenage children

With the average age of first-time mothers in England and Wales now nearing 30, the chances are most women's menopause will coincide with the hormonal whirlwind of puberty.[68]

Both of you are on a hormonal rollercoaster: like you, your teenager is coping with changes to their body, mood swings and could be hit by low self-esteem. A little bit of tact and a lot of communication can help to avoid your menopause and their teenage years being played out to the sound of slamming doors and stony silences.

Remember to include your teenager in discussions about your menopause. Tell them what is happening and why. Understandably, my daughters constantly hear about my work so now know a considerable amount about the menopause, but they are in the minority.

For such a crucial stage in every woman's life, menopause education is woefully lacking in our schools. While they have (quite rightly) been taught about sex and contraception, the only fact my two teenage daughters have been told about the menopause in school is that it is when periods stop. If only it was that simple.

Your teenagers will be sensitive to, and maybe alarmed at, seeing you go through physical and emotional changes (don't forget it was my middle daughter's comments about my moods that helped me realise I was perimenopausal). Reassurance that your menopause is entirely normal and natural will help allay any worries they may have.

Recently, my two older daughters were talking about how dreadful I was before I started HRT. They admitted that

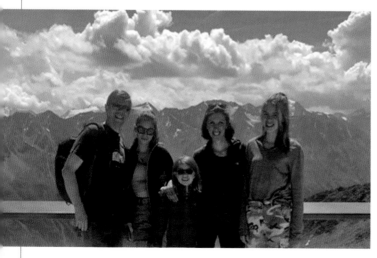

← Keeping communication channels open between you and your children is so important.

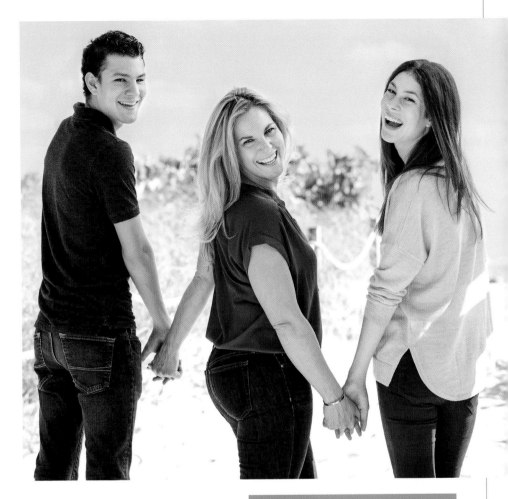

they were so worried about my moods at times they feared our family would break up. Looking back, while it is easy to make light of the memory slips, forgetting birthdays or where I had put my car keys, it is frightening to think the effect my symptoms were having on my family unit.

That's why communication is so key. But you need to pick your moments when to talk to each other. Ten minutes before you leave for work and your teenager is rushing to school may not be the best time to have a heart to heart.

For more information

Relate has a great section on its website on communicating with teenagers: www.relate.org.uk

The Royal College of Psychiatrists has a page on surviving adolescence for parents and carers on the young people's mental health section of their website: www,rcpsych.ac.uk

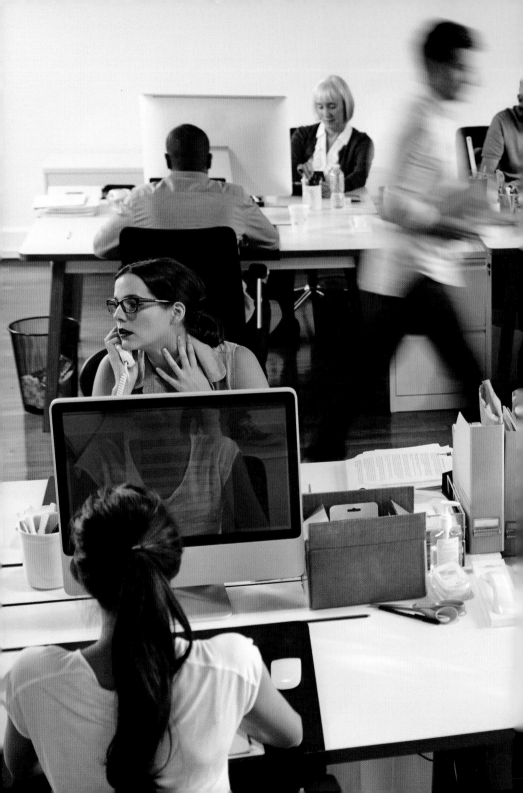

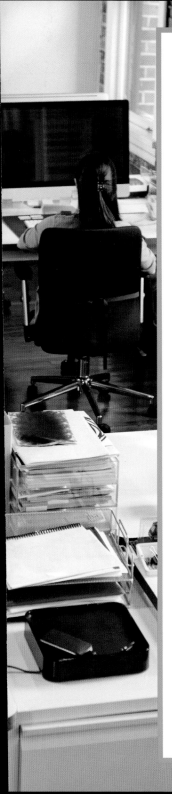

Chapter 7
Menopause and work

Women are working later in life than ever before, with an estimated 4.3 million women over 50 currently employed in the UK.[70] Yet despite women now making up half of the UK's labour force – and many going through their menopause during their working lives – the menopause remains an overlooked issue in too many organisations. With some practical changes and emotional support in place, your menopause needn't be a barrier to a long and fulfilling career.

In this chapter, I will be covering your rights in the workplace and how to get the support you need during your perimenopause and menopause, including:

◆ How to broach the subject with your manager
◆ Getting the adjustments you need
◆ Alternative working arrangements
◆ Creating a support network with colleagues, and coping strategies.

There is also advice for employers on making their workplace menopause friendly – and why one size doesn't fit all.

Menopause and your career

Try mentioning the word 'menopause' at work and it is likely to stun people into silence or cause an embarrassing giggle at a hormonal woman's expense.

Employers are (quite rightly) sympathetic towards pregnant women who feel tired, or to a new parent suffering from sleepless nights. Sadly, that same sympathy is not always extended to women who have disturbed sleep or a host of other symptoms because of their menopause.

A 2017 government-commissioned review into the effects of menopausal symptoms on women's working lives found that, unlike pregnancy or maternity, the menopause is not well understood or provided for in workplace culture, policies or training.[70] The review also found that attitudes of some managers and work colleagues towards menopausal women (or mid-life women in general) showed a 'lack of knowledge, understanding and support indicating widespread gendered ageism'.

So it is no wonder the vast majority of women I treat feel uncomfortable talking about their menopause at work. In my career I have helped women including barristers, nurses, doctors, hairdressers, dog groomers, accountants and athletes. I hear time and time again that many women feel they have no

option but to reduce their hours, change roles or even quit work altogether because they struggle with symptoms. Others feel acute embarrassment about their symptoms, or suffer a crisis of confidence, meaning they won't put themselves forward for promotion.

Research shows that the more troublesome menopausal symptoms are, the less engaged women feel at work. They feel less satisfied with their job, have lower levels of commitment, and have a greater intention to quit their job altogether. Studies also show that menopausal symptoms can have a significant impact on attendance and performance. Some women can be misdiagnosed as suffering from mental ill health or other conditions, and the detrimental impact symptoms have can be wrongly seen as a performance issue.

It really doesn't have to be like that. There are some signs that governments are finally taking the menopause seriously. Conservative MP Rachel Maclean, who has long campaigned for greater menopause awareness, held a debate on the NHS and the menopause in early 2019, and won backing for her campaign from the prime minister. The Scottish government has also pledged better support for menopausal women in the workplace.[71] And in recent years more organisations are finally wising up to the fact that it pays to be menopause friendly – and that it means more than installing a few token desk fans to combat hot flushes.

> ## Did you know?
>
> *One in ten women have considered giving up work due to their menopausal symptoms.*[72]

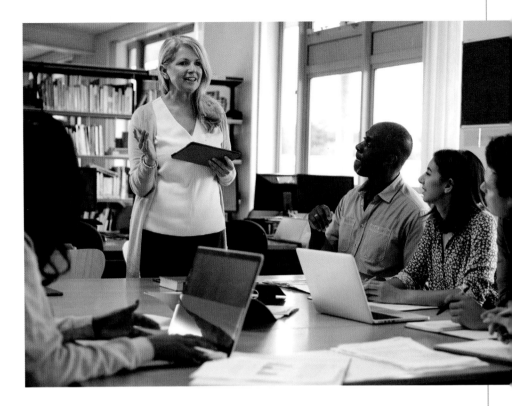

I have seen first-hand from my work advising large organisations such as West Midlands Police and West Midlands Fire Service that if the menopause is handled correctly and sensitively, it helps to reduce absenteeism and allows women to talk more openly about their concerns with colleagues and managers.

There IS something you can do about it

Your menopause is a completely normal life event. It is not an illness or a medical condition. Yet this means that the symptoms of your menopause – particularly the psychological ones – are all too often under recognised, undervalued and not taken seriously enough. If this rings true in your workplace, then it is time

↑ Your career should not have to suffer because of your menopause.

for your employer to put things right. While no specific legislation exists to cover the menopause at work, employers do have a responsibility to ensure the health and safety of all employees.

Frustratingly few workplaces have a menopause policy in place. If this is the case where you work, then a good starting point is to take in a copy of guidance on the menopause and the workplace from the Faculty of Occupational Medicine. These guidelines, the key points of which I will cover in this chapter, provide clear recommendations about working conditions for menopausal women experiencing troublesome symptoms.

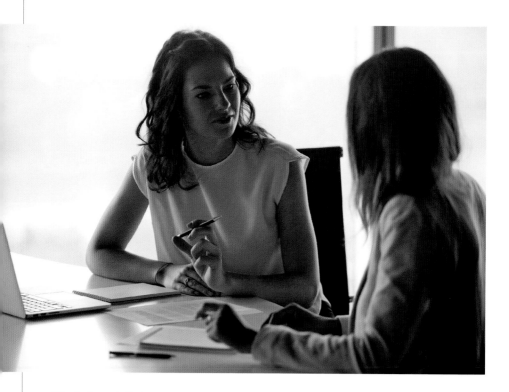

First step: talk to your line manager

It is no surprise that so many of us find work difficult due to symptoms of our menopause. Poor concentration, tiredness, poor memory, depression, feeling low, reduced confidence, sleep deprivation and hot flushes are often cited as symptoms that can really take their toll in the workplace. We undertook a survey of 335 women in mid-life working for West Midlands Police and the results were presented at the International Menopause Society conference. Results from this survey revealed that 82% felt their menopausal symptoms had a negative impact on their working life.

Disclosing your menopausal symptoms to your managers and colleagues is of course a matter of personal choice. Yet

↑ Being open about your symptoms could help secure the workplace changes you need.

being open about how you feel, rather than keeping quiet about your symptoms, can be a crucial first step in securing the support you need. First, ask your manager for a meeting. This is a chance to outline your symptoms and request changes to your daily work that could help.

Before the meeting, take some time to compile a list of the symptoms you are experiencing and have a few concrete examples of how they might be affecting your work. Do long conference calls in stifling rooms trigger a hot flush? Has there been a particular task or project that you have struggled with because of poor concentration?

Be honest – and don't suffer in silence

University of Nottingham research published by the British Occupational Health Research Foundation into the experience of women working through their menopause found that where women had taken time off work to deal with their symptoms, only half had disclosed the real reasons for absence to their line managers.[73] Never feel embarrassed to ask for help. You are not being unreasonable for asking for changes to the way you work, or to want your workplace to be more open about the menopause.

Many studies show that there is a long-established link between employee good health and workplace performance. The general hypothesis is that the healthier and happier people are, the more productive they are likely to be in the workplace. Regardless of whether your symptoms are forcing you to take time off, your menopause needs to be a key consideration in your overall health and happiness at work.

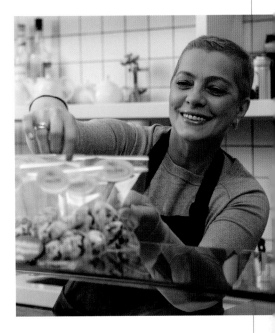

Don't want to be 'managed' through your menopause? Here are some proactive, practical solutions

We know that there is often more to your menopause than hot flushes, but does your employer? If no clear menopause policy exists in your workplace, then try to

Manager unsympathetic? Then speak to someone else

If you feel uncomfortable raising the issue with your manager, you are not alone. Only 28% of the women who took part in the West Midlands Police survey disclosed their menopausal symptoms to their line managers. Reasons for not speaking up included a fear of perceived incompetence, with one woman saying she tried to 'cope alone so no one can say that I am not fit to do my duties', while another didn't want to talk to their manager because 'he's a younger man and won't understand'. Yet it was encouraging that 69% of women who did talk to their line managers found it a positive experience.

If you find your manager is unapproachable, don't be put off. The Faculty of Occupational Medicine suggests making an appointment with human resources, or even speaking to another manager who you feel more comfortable with.

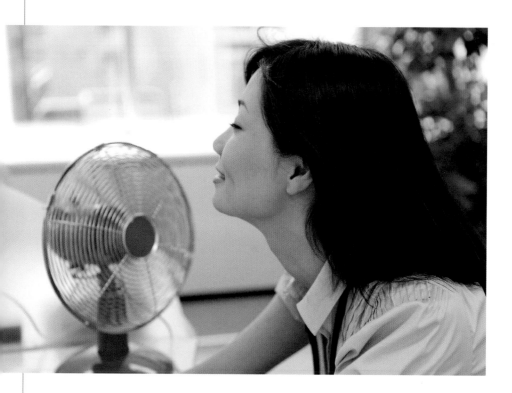

A desktop fan could help with hot flushes.

be as specific as possible in what changes (known as adjustments) you might need to be happier and more productive. This conversation might be one you can have with your line manager, but you could speak to human resources to ask for an assessment. If an occupational health service is available, you could also ask to speak to them. Here are some changes the Faculty of Occupational Medicine suggests employers should consider:

◆ Feeling the heat? Then ask to move desks. Employers should review workplace temperature and ventilation to see how they might be adapted. This could include providing you with a desktop fan or making sure your workstation is near an opening window or away from a heat source.[74]

◆ Provide access to cold drinking water in all work situations.
◆ Access to wash room facilities.
◆ Time out: if your role is public facing, you could ask for access to a quiet room for a short break (for example, to manage a severe hot flush). A quiet space would also be beneficial if your job involves a lot of standing. On the other hand, if your job is desk-based or very sedentary, then space to move about should be considered.
◆ Wear a uniform? You can ask employers to be flexible in allowing you to remove neckties or jackets, and also provide changing facilities.

Flexible working: how to ask for it

You may find that changing your working pattern could help to alleviate some of your most troublesome symptoms. For example, a later starting time could be beneficial if you are suffering from sleep problems, or working from home in a quiet space when you have a deadline could combat poor concentration. Many women working for West Midlands Police have been given adjusted hours, which has made a real difference to them. Some have told me that having an understanding boss who can be flexible to a changing work pattern depending on symptoms can make a huge difference. Some women have changed their roles in the organisation which means they can do a different job much easier without being judged differently.

Flexible working could include working from home, working part-time or switching to compressed hours. According to government guidance (www.gov.uk/flexible-working/applying-for-flexible-working), as long as you have worked continuously for the same employer for 26 weeks, you have the right to request flexible working. The basic steps are:

1 You write to your employer.
2 Your employer considers the request and makes a decision, usually within three months.
3 If your employer agrees to the request, they must change the terms and conditions in your contract.
4 If they refuse, they must write to you giving business reasons for the refusal. You may be able to complain to an employment tribunal if you disagree with the outcome.
5 Note that rules around flexible working are different in Northern Ireland.

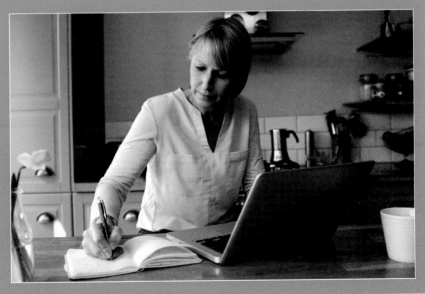

Self-help: tips to manage your menopause at work

Your menopause often occurs at an important point in your career, so it can be easy to blame some symptoms on the stresses of everyday life.

You could be coping with a very busy period at work, as well as juggling caring responsibilities for children, parents, a partner or even grandchildren. But one thing you should never underestimate is the huge hormonal upheaval you experience during your perimenopause and menopause, and the effect that can have on how you handle work and your relationship with your colleagues.

Environmental factors such as stuffy offices and general workplace stress arising from deadlines and office politics can make menopausal symptoms worse. A Trades Union Congress survey of 500 safety representatives revealed that half of respondents thought the workplace made menopausal symptoms worse.[75]

In addition to asking for greater support and adjustments from your employer, some of the treatments and coping strategies we have discussed earlier in this manual can be of real benefit in the workplace. Discuss your treatment options with your doctor or health professional to get the best treatment for you. Please don't needlessly struggle on. Many women do not realise how effective HRT can be at dramatically improving their symptoms and quality of life, which in turn means you function better at work. The Faculty of Occupational Health also recommends talking to colleagues about your menopause. Bottling things up or concealing your symptoms for fear of looking unprofessional or not up to the job, only piles on more stress, making your symptoms worse. It also suggests making any necessary lifestyle changes, such as more exercise, stopping smoking or losing weight if you need to. CBT could be worth exploring to combat anxiety and low mood.

How to talk to your colleagues
I'm not suggesting you call a departmental meeting and launch into a PowerPoint

Three-minute stress buster

This simple breathing exercise can help to relieve feelings of stress or anxiety. Try to do this exercise for three to five minutes every day – once you get the hang of it you could even do it at your desk.

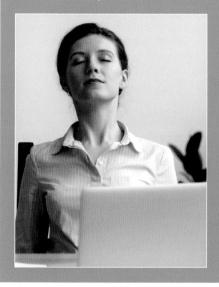

1 Sit on a chair and make yourself comfortable, ensuring that your clothing is not restricting your breathing.

2 Remain seated and place your arms on the chair arms, feet hip-width apart.

3 Breathe in through your nose and out through your mouth, allowing the breath to flow deep into your stomach.

4 Breathe in gently, steadily counting from one to five. Let the breath flow out gently, again counting from one to five, and repeat for three to five minutes.

← Setting aside just a few minutes a day to breathe deeply could help ease stress.

presentation of your medical records, but it may help to be upfront with colleagues so they know what you are going through. Keep it informal: suggest going out for lunch with your closest colleagues and let them know what symptoms you are coping with. Crucial to this conversation is clearly communicating what they can do to help, for example no longer scheduling nine o'clock meetings if you are struggling with insomnia or pointing out that plugging in a heater right by your desk isn't helpful.

Build an emotional support network. Watch and listen for your colleagues' reactions. You may find that others are menopausal too. If so, build your own support network. Why not get out of the office by going for a regular lunchtime stroll, to give yourself time away from your desk and a chance to talk to people who understand what you are going through. You might even find that some colleagues have a partner who is going through her menopause and may also welcome the opportunity to talk.

Consider starting a menopause group either for women to meet at or via social media. This has worked really well for many organisations I have worked with and women feel supported even if they do this in an anonymous way using the internet.

Tackling brain fog and memory problems

Many women who come to my menopause and wellbeing centre talk primarily about their struggles with physical symptoms such as hot flushes or night sweats, but digging a little deeper I usually find that it is the cognitive and psychological changes that have the biggest impact on their home and working lives.

Poor concentration, memory problems and verbal slips are classic symptoms of the perimenopause and menopause. That's because estrogen and testosterone often have an important role to play on cognition and memory, so when these levels reduce, we feel the effects. And it is symptoms like these that have caused many successful and high-powered business women to give up work either because they simply can't cope any more or are convinced they are losing their mind. I see many women who are worried they have dementia as they have a worsening memory and are constantly forgetting things. Finding you've left your car keys in the fridge might be funny; not so amusing when you forget a big work meeting.

Brain fog, or an inability to think clearly, is another very common symptom. Women have told me that their brains feel like cotton wool and they find it very difficult to absorb information. This can be a challenge with a hectic job, but it can also affect simple tasks such as reading a book or listening to the radio. I know all too well what it is like to cope with brain fog while at work. I found I was struggling to remember patients' names, constantly rechecking prescriptions to ensure I had not made any mistakes. I felt permanently tired and was often irritable with some of my colleagues.

As ever, consult with your doctor or another health professional on getting the right treatment for you, but you could also give the following a try:

Make a note of it:
If your memory and concentration is an issue, keep a work diary on your phone to set reminders for important dates. If you have a meeting coming up, prepare some notecards in advance to serve as a visual prompt.

A walk in the park:
Use your break to rest and eat, not to rush out to the shops or for online banking. A 2017 study of 50 workers found those who had a 15-minute lunchtime walk in the park or engaged in a relaxation exercise had better levels of concentration and reduced stress in the afternoon.[76]

Plan your day:
Morning tends to be when we are at our most focused, so tackle big projects before lunch. Save more monotonous tasks that may not require as much concentration (such as reading emails) for later in the day.

A healthy desk set-up

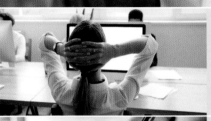

Avoid hot flush triggers like caffeine, particularly before an important meeting. Sip water instead.

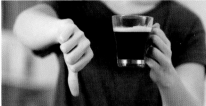

Take regular screen breaks (away from your desk if possible) to rest your eyes and retain mental focus. The Health and Safety Executive recommends short, frequent breaks of five to ten minutes every hour on non-screen work rather than longer breaks every few hours.[77]

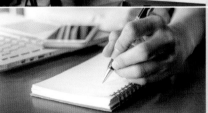

Beat brain fog by making notes of important tasks or dates to refer to when your concentration wavers.

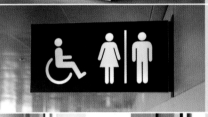

Ask to move desks to be nearer to a bathroom if you need to.

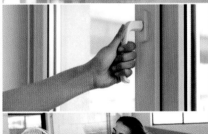

Position your desk near a window to get some ventilation and natural light to help regulate your body clock.

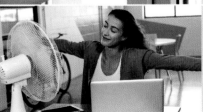

Have an electric or handheld fan close by to help cool down quickly. Wear loose layers (preferably breathable cotton) so you can easily take some clothes off if you overheat.

Are you an employer? Here's what you need to be doing

Research has shown that (understandably) many women do not feel comfortable formally discussing their specific menopausal symptoms with an organisation, nor do they want to feel 'managed' through their menopause in any way.

However, many women also feel that if their organisation took a proactive approach and the cultural perception of menopause shifted, then this could have a significant effect on their work and career prospects.

From my day to day work at my clinic and through my work with organisations like the West Midlands Police, it is very clear that women do not want to simply be offered fans or to work with better air conditioning. What they want, and deserve, is for other people to appreciate and understand the numerous symptoms that can affect women at this stage of their lives.

The sooner employers see that, just like pregnancy, the menopause is an occupational health issue, the better. If you don't have a menopause policy, get one drawn up as soon as possible. Employers should be supporting menopausal women as part of a holistic approach to employee health and wellbeing. Get a copy of the Faculty of Occupational Health guidance. The Chartered Institute of Personnel and Development has also published free guidance on managing the menopause in the workplace.

Above all, remember every woman's menopause is different: some women have mild symptoms, others endure symptoms for several years. Listen carefully to each woman and be prepared to tailor any support.

Your policy could include:

◆ Menopause awareness training: training can help employees (female and male) understand the basics of the menopause, issues that can arise and what they can do to help. Use humour to make training a positive experience and to get the message across. West Midlands Police enlisted the help of Laughology, a training organisation founded by a comedian which uses the psychology of humour and laughter, to deliver training workshops on the menopause (www.laughology.co.uk). Another organisation is Talking Menopause, which was set up by former My Menopause Doctor business manager Sarah Davies and Lynda Bailey, a former West Midlands Police inspector. It has delivered menopause training to police forces, fire services and multinationals (www. talkingmenopause.co.uk).

◆ Clear, easily accessible information on the menopause: if you have a work intranet site, create a menopause page, with information on causes, symptoms, treatments, and coping strategies. Include links to further medical advice (such as the NHS Choices website) and contact details for human resources or occupational health.

◆ Webchat/FAQs: regular webchats or myth-busting sessions with a healthcare professional who is experienced in helping women through the menopause will give staff a trusted source of advice. This may also be a helpful tool for employees whose partners are going through the menopause.

- Set up a menopause forum: give employees time and space to meet with others to share experiences, swap suggestions for ways of coping and as a place to raise issues for employers to consider. One woman who attended a similar forum at West Midlands Police said of her experience: 'I attend the menopause support group and what a fabulous group of ladies they are. It's the first time I've felt that everything has fallen into place for me.'

- Create a reasonable adjustment passport: these passports are a record of adjustments agreed between an employee and their manager because of a health condition, impairment or disability. The purpose of the passport is so everyone is clear what changes have been agreed, and to reduce the need for reassessment every time an employee changes role or is assigned a new manager.[78] West Midlands Police have adopted a similar passport for women with menopausal symptoms, which is a fantastic idea – women don't have to repeat their story and symptoms every time they move department, and their adjustments are already on paper.

- Be flexible: be open to any flexible working requests where possible. Allowing a woman to change her working hours or even work from home could make all the difference in her tackling her menopausal symptoms or feeling like she has no choice but to leave.

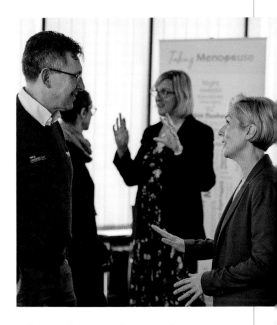

⬆ Listen to what your employees expect from you, and be flexible.

For more information

Chartered Institute of Personnel and Development: www.cipd.co.uk

Faculty of Occupational Medicine: www.fom.ac.uk

Flexible working: www.gov.uk/flexible-working

NHS Choices menopause information: www.nhs.uk/conditions/menopause

Talking Menopause: www.talkingmenopause.co.uk

Postscript
New beginnings – life after menopause

'I've regained my husband, sanity and family. I'm able to cuddle my granddaughter. I'm beginning to live again.'

These powerful words are from a patient who, prior to coming to my clinic, had been suffering from low mood, anxiety and suicidal thoughts for a number of years. She had been prescribed antidepressants and even electroconvulsive therapy by psychiatrists, all to no avail. Yet her life was transformed by the right treatment (in her case HRT) and her inspiring story is proof that no one should have to suffer their menopause in silence. With the right advice, support and treatment, you can get back to living the life you want and deserve.

I hope the information, treatment advice, good lifestyle habits and coping strategies you've picked up throughout this manual will see you through into the next stage of your life: your postmenopause. We women spend on average a third of our lives postmenopausal,[9] so let's make them some of our best years.

Are we nearly there yet?
One of the most common questions I get asked by women in my clinic and on social media is 'When will my menopause be over?' Sadly, the answer is not as simple as we would like. The average length of your menopause is about four years after your last period, but one in ten women can experience symptoms for up to 12 years.[8]

It would be helpful here to remind ourselves of the different stages of your menopause:

- Perimenopause is the time before your menopause when you start to experience symptoms because of changing hormone levels.
- Menopause is when you haven't had a period for one year.
- Postmenopause refers to the time *after* you have not had a period for 12 consecutive months.

How will I know when my menopause is ending?
An estimated 80% of women will be postmenopausal by the age of 54.[79] Thankfully, many women who suffer

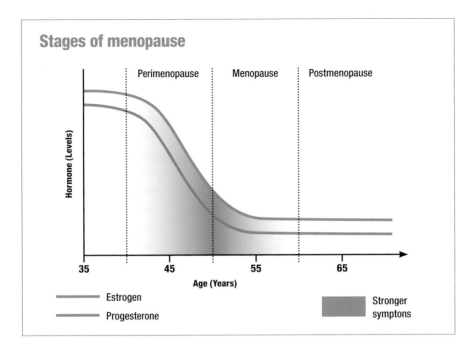

Stages of menopause

Perimenopause · Menopause · Postmenopause

Hormone (Levels)

Age (Years)

35 · 45 · 55 · 65

Estrogen
Progesterone

Stronger
symptons

from hot flushes and night sweats find they get better with time, but other symptoms may present themselves, such as trouble sleeping, anxiety and low energy levels. Vaginal dryness is a very common problem that persists and often worsens postmenopause, affecting more than half of women after their menopause.[80] Symptoms often worsen with time as once the tissues are thin they do not repair and regenerate without estrogen. Remember, there are a range of treatments, both hormonal and non-hormonal, that can ease symptoms.

There are two new treatments that can help post-menopausal women with moderate to severe symptoms of vulvovaginal atrophy – which includes dryness and soreness in and around the vagina, and pain during intercourse. The first is Ospemifene, an oral, non-hormonal treatment taken once a day. It belongs to a group of drugs known as

selective estrogen receptor modulators, which means it stimulates the receptor for estrogen in some tissues in the body such as the vagina, helping to reverse symptoms of vulvovaginal atrophy. Ospemifene could be an option for women for women who find using topical creams or vaginal tablets difficult to use.

The second is Intrarosa, a vaginal pessary available on prescription from late 2019. Intrarosa contains an active ingredient called prasterone, which is converted into estrogens and androgens in the vagina and improves the tissues in and around the vagina. Trials have shown it helps reduce signs of thinning and has a modest reduction in pain during intercourse.

On a positive note, some women find that their energy levels improve postmenopause, and some women do find that their sex drive improves.

I'm on HRT: when should I stop taking it?

There is no set length of time you should take HRT for – my oldest patient is 93 years old. Menopause guidelines both at home and abroad clearly state that HRT may be taken for as long as necessary and as long as the benefits outweigh any risks. The dose of estrogen usually decreases with age as the body requires less. Some women only want to take HRT for a short time to help with their symptoms, while others decide to take it for longer to help with their mood, energy and concentration and also to improve their future health. This is because taking HRT reduces future risk of heart disease, osteoporosis and diabetes.

Staying safe

Note that even though the chances of getting pregnant after 55 are extremely slim, don't forget that you'll still need to practise safe sex and use a condom to protect yourself from sexually transmitted infections.

If you are taking HRT then you should be seeing a health professional for an annual review, but if you have any concerns about any medication you may be taking for your symptoms, make an appointment. It's key you have a discussion with a health professional about what is right for your individual circumstances.

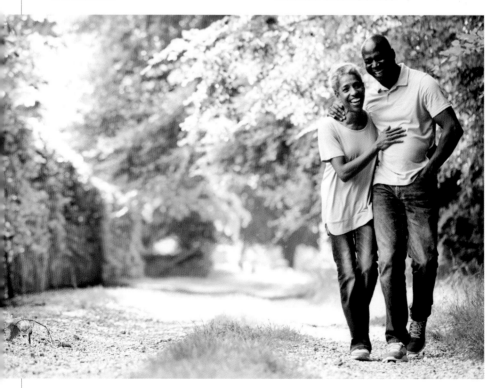

Good habits to last a lifetime

Even if your menopause was relatively symptom free, low hormones will still have an impact on your postmenopausal health. Low hormones put you at greater risk of conditions such as osteoporosis and cardiovascular disease, but the good news is that treatment and a healthy diet and lifestyle can help mitigate some of those risks.

Ageing can raise the risk of certain cancers, so it is also really important that you attend regular screening appointments, such as breast and cervical screening (more information can be found at www.nhs.uk/conditions/nhs-screening).

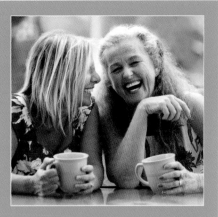

Take charge of your postmenopause diet

Osteoporosis is a key concern postmenopause. About 10% of a woman's bone mass is lost in the first five years of the menopause and one in two postmenopausal women develop osteoporosis, so eat a balanced diet with plenty of calcium and vitamin D to aid calcium absorption.

Keep active

Exercise boosts your mood, keeps bones healthy and reduces the risk of high blood pressure and cardiovascular disease. Aim for 30 minutes of moderate exercise, five times a week, and strength exercise on two or more days a week. Incorporate some weight-bearing exercises to help keep your bones strong. Remember that doing just a few minutes' exercise is better than doing nothing at all.

Take time out

Your body has been through so many changes in recent years, and it is bound to have taken a toll on you physically and mentally. Be proud of yourself and take some time for you that makes you happy – spending time with loved ones, catching up with friends or even taking some time to do some breathing for relaxation for a few minutes at the end of each day.

Above all, keeping talking

I'm passionate about the fact that no woman should have to go through her menopause alone. You are now knowledgeable, so pass that knowledge on. Talk to your loved ones at home, your managers, your colleagues. Point them in the direction of credible information sources about the menopause. Most importantly, talk to your female friends, daughters and granddaughters about your experiences so they know it's fine to talk about their perimenopause and menopause when the time comes. We will never be able to break the taboo of menopause unless we ourselves talk about it, so let's make that change now!

Appendix I
The Greene Climacteric Scale

Symptoms	Not at all 0	A little 1	Quite a bit 2	Extremely 3	Comment
Heart beating quickly or strongly					
Feeling tense or nervous					
Difficulty in sleeping					
Excitable					
Attacks of anxiety, panic					
Difficulty in concentrating					
Feeling tired or lacking in energy					
Loss of interest in most things					
Feeling unhappy or depressed					
Crying spells					
Irritability					

Please indicate the extent to which you are bothered at the moment by any of these symptoms by placing a tick in the appropriate box.

Symptoms *continued*	Not at all 0	A little 1	Quite a bit 2	Extremely 3	Comment
Feeling dizzy or faint					
Pressure or tightness in head					
Parts of body feel numb					
Headaches					
Muscle and joint pains					
Loss of feeling in hands or feet					
Breathing difficulties					
Hot flushes					
Sweating at night					
Loss of interest in sex					
SCORE					

Appendix II
Tips for your loved ones

Communication is so important during your menopause, but at times it can be hard to put how you are feeling into words. Why not get the conversation started by sharing the following hints and tips with your male partner and/or your children. Leave a copy of this manual, or suggest they have a read (of this appendix, at least) during a quiet moment – and offer to have a discussion afterwards in case they have any questions.

For your partner

It is important to remember that your partner's menopause is not an illness, but a completely normal stage of her life. Of course that doesn't always mean that her menopause will be a breeze and, as a partner, it can be a time of change and uncertainty for you too.

A lot of women bring their partners along to appointments at my clinic for moral support. Despairing partners tell me how they find it hard to recognise the person they fell in love with and would do anything to help them get better. Many say they had no idea the menopause could have such a physical and psychological impact on their loved one, and that they have nowhere to turn to for information or advice. I hope these tips will make the menopause easier for her and you.

Don't be left in the dark

Read up on your partner's menopause; how it happens, why it happens and symptoms she may be experiencing. Read Chapter 1 of this manual, the NICE menopause guidelines or the NHS Choices website.

Hormone changes can have a powerful impact on your partner's body and cause a range of symptoms. She will by no means have every symptom, but it is good to be aware of common symptoms that could be down to her menopause. Be mindful that not every symptom is physical and that some symptoms can exacerbate others, like night sweats and poor sleep.

Ask questions to help prepare for what is ahead, why she is feeling the way she is feeling and how you can best support her.

Be patient

If she has forgotten an important event, or her mind seems elsewhere, it isn't because she's not interested. Memory problems and poor concentration are common in perimenopause and menopause. This is because as estrogen and testosterone (hormones which fluctuate at this time) play an important role in cognition and memory.

If her tossing and turning is keeping you awake at night, it could be down to night sweats, urinary problems or even stress causing poor sleep and early morning waking.

Resist the urge to bite back

Falling estrogen levels can commonly cause mood changes, leading to anger, irritability, frustration or tearfulness. If you find yourself at the receiving end, don't shout back. Take a moment to collect your thoughts and try to see it from her perspective. If you were suffering from hot

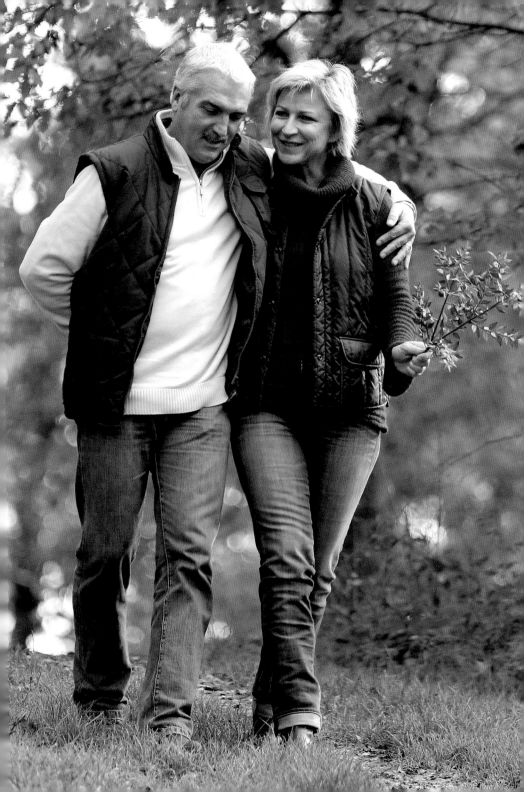

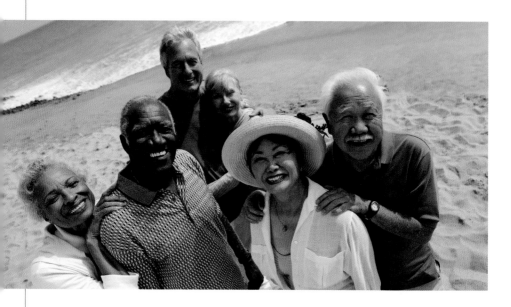

flushes, had aching joints or hadn't slept properly in days, you would be feeling exasperated too. Listen, acknowledge her frustrations and talk things through.

Take an interest

Menopause is not just 'women's business'. Your partner's health and wellbeing impacts you and your wider family. Offer practical support, such as helping to research treatment and coping strategies. Offer to accompany her to any medical appointments, but don't be offended if she prefers to go alone. At the very least, remember when she has an appointment so you can have a debrief afterwards.

… but don't take over

No woman wants to feel 'managed' through their menopause. Be tactful but resist the urge to take over.

Sex may be the last thing on her mind

Changing hormones can lead to a lower libido, and vaginal dryness and irritation can make sex painful. Your partner may also be feeling self-conscious about changes to her body.

Rethink your social life

In the past, you may have enjoyed winding down as a couple over a bottle of wine. But alcohol, caffeine and spicy foods can trigger hot flushes, so these might not feel like the treats they once did. Your partner may not find the same enjoyment she once did in some activities you did together, so think of some alternatives. A weekend stroll will give you some breathing space away from home life, and count as exercise too. Or how about some escapism with a trip to the cinema (the air conditioning may be a welcome relief from hot flushes too)?

Take some time out for yourself

It can be difficult to see your partner having a hard time, so talk to family, talk to friends – they may be going through the same with their own partners. Menopause Cafés are open to men too.

My mum's menopause: tips for teenagers

It's a time of change

During puberty, your body and mind are going through a lot of changes. The NHS website Health for Teens is a really good source of information (www.healthforteens.co.uk).

Levels of your hormones, the chemical messengers that travel through our body, change during puberty, affecting your growth, development and mood. And just like in puberty, your mum's menopause also means she is also going through some physical and emotional changes because of hormones.

Do your homework

Not in the school or college sense but do your menopause homework. Ask your mum questions about her menopause, what it is and how it makes her feel and act. If you've noticed your mum acting differently recently, talking about it could help you understand why.

Don't worry

You may be finding things difficult at the moment, but these times will pass. Like puberty, your mum's menopause is completely natural and a normal part of being a woman.

Keep talking

The most important thing you can do is keeping talking to each other. If it feels like there's never the right moment to speak to your mum, then why not put pen to paper?

Talking to your siblings and friends can help too. You might also find that your friends' mums are going through the same thing – in fact, my daughter correctly guessed that a school friend's mum was having hot flushes and was menopausal after hearing how she was having baths in the middle of the night to cool down!

Offer a helping hand

Your mum might be feeling overwhelmed at the moment, with physical aches and pains and emotions, as well as her work and family life. Is there anything that you and the rest of the family can do to help her out?

Look after your body and mind

Eating a balanced diet is important for both you and your mum at this time, so you could try researching healthy recipes that you can make together.

Exercise is also really important too – you should be getting at least 60 minutes a day of exercise to help build stronger bones and muscles and boost your self-esteem. Your mum should be getting lots of exercise too (about 30 minutes a day, five times a week) so why not look at some classes or activities that you could try together, like swimming, walking or yoga.

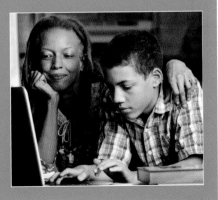

Cancer and the menopause: what you need to know

Although most women will go through their menopause naturally, certain treatments for cancer can trigger an early menopause.

Going through an early menopause as a result of cancer treatment can be distressing: you may feel isolated and confused about the changes.

The onset of an early menopause can be sudden, and symptoms such as hot flushes, vaginal dryness and mood changes can be hard to cope with alongside your cancer diagnosis and treatment.

That is why it is so important to be prepared, and to ask for support when you need it.

Why can my cancer treatment affect when I go through the menopause?

Certain cancer treatments can stop the ovaries from working properly and bring about an earlier menopause.

These include:

♦ Surgery involving the ovaries, such as an oophorectomy, where one or both ovaries are removed. You may also have one or both of your ovaries removed during a hysterectomy (an operation where your uterus is removed). Women can still experience an early menopause if they have had a hysterectomy without their ovaries being removed
♦ Radiotherapy to the pelvic area
♦ Certain types of chemotherapy drugs to treat cancer

If your menopause occurs between the ages of 40 and 45, it is known as an early menopause.

If it occurs before the age of 40, it is known as premature ovarian insufficiency (POI).

Will my menopause be temporary or permanent?

This is dependent on a number of factors, including your age and the type of cancer treatment you are having.

If you have an oophorectomy or a hysterectomy where both ovaries are removed then you will have your menopause immediately, regardless of age. If one of your ovaries is left intact after an oophorectomy (or both are intact after a hysterectomy), there's a chance that you'll experience the menopause within five years of having surgery.

The menopause after pelvic radiotherapy or chemotherapy could be temporary or permanent. This usually depends on how close you are to the age of your natural menopause, and the dose of radiation or type of drugs used.

What symptoms can I expect?

If your menopause has been triggered by treatment for cancer, your symptoms will be similar to those of a natural menopause.

However, vaginal dryness and recurrent urinary tract infections (UTIs) can be more common in women going through their menopause as a result of cancer treatment. It can be a particular problem for women who take Tamoxifen, a hormonal therapy drug use to treat some types of cancers including breast cancer.

Long term health problems which can arise from your menopause

An early menopause can put you at risk of various health conditions at an earlier age, such as osteoporosis and cardiovascular disease.

Will my fertility be affected?

This depends on your individual circumstances such as your age and the type of treatment you have.

NICE menopause guidelines clearly state that women who are likely to go through menopause as a result of medical or surgical treatment should be offered support.

You should also be given information about menopause before you have treatment and ideally should be referred to a healthcare professional with expertise in menopause.

You should expect to discuss risk of early menopause, how your fertility might be affected, common menopausal symptoms, longer-term health implications of menopause and advice about contraception.

Is HRT suitable for me?

If your cancer is not hormone-dependant (such as certain types of breast cancers) then you should be able to take HRT. Speak to a health professional, ideally a doctor who specialises in the menopause, about your individual circumstances so you can make an informed decision.

Remember that you should be given information about the impact of an early menopause before cancer treatment begins; you should not have to wait until your menopause symptoms become unbearable before seeking help.

If you are taking HRT and feel like your symptoms aren't improving within a few months, speak to a health professional. Going through your menopause at a younger age often means your body's requirement for hormones is greater compared to older women.

It may be that your HRT dose is too low - many young women actually need two or even three times more HRT than the average dose given to older women – so your dosage or delivery method may need adjusting.

Other treatments

There are some alternative prescription medications that can be prescribed for symptoms if you are unable or choose not to take HRT.

These include some types of antidepressants such as citalopram or venlafaxine can improve hot flushes, but they can have side effects such as nausea and low libido. There are also lifestyle changes that can make a positive difference, such as changing your diet and exercising. Some women also find their symptoms improve by changing their cancer treatment – for example taking tamoxifen rather than an aromatase inhibitor. You should always speak to your oncologist for advice about changing or stopping any cancer treatments.

Where can I go to for more advice?

This may feel like a very isolating time, but there are a number of sources of advice for women coping with cancer and their menopause, including:

◆ The Eve Appeal is a charity funding research into and raising awareness of womb, ovarian, cervical, vulval and vaginal cancers www.eveappeal.org.uk
◆ Daisy Network is a charity for women affected by POI www.daisynetwork.org.uk
◆ Macmillan Cancer Support www.macmillan.org.uk
◆ Cancer Research UK www.cancerresearchuk.org
◆ My Menopause Doctor www.menopausedoctor.co.uk
◆ NICE information for women having treatment likely to cause menopause www.tinyurl.com/NICE-menopause-treatment

References

1. Cumming GP, Currie H, Morris E, et al. (2015) The need to do better: are we still letting our patients down and at what cost? *Post Reproductive Health* 21(2): 56–62.
2. Nuffield Health (2014, 17 October) One in four with menopause symptoms concerned about ability to cope with life. www.nuffieldhealth. com/article/one-in-four-with-menopause-symptoms-concerned-about-ability-to-cope-with-life.
3. NHS Choices (2018) Menopause: Overview. www.nhs.uk/conditions/menopause
4. Daisy Network (2019) What is POI? www. daisynetwork.org/about-poi/what-is-poi
5. NHS Choices (2019) Hysterectomy: Considerations. www.nhs.uk/conditions/ hysterectomy/considerations
6. National Institute for Health and Care Excellence (2015) Menopause as a result of medical treatment, in *Menopause Diagnosis and Management: Information for the Public*. London: NICE. www.nice.org.uk/guidance/ ng23/ifp/chapter/Menopause-as-a-result-of-medical-treatment
7. National Institute for Health and Care Excellence (2015) Diagnosis of perimenopause and menopause, in *Menopause: Diagnosis and Management*. London: NICE. www.nice.org.uk/ guidance/ng23/chapter/ Recommendations#diagnosis-of-perimenopause-and-menopause
8. Avis NE, Crawford SL, Greendale G, et al. (2015) Duration of menopausal vasomotor symptoms over the menopause transition. *JAMA Internal Medicine* 175(4): 531–39.
9. Currie H, Abernethy K, Gray S (2017) *Vision for Menopause Care in the UK*. Marlow: British Menopause Society. https://thebms.org.uk/ wp-content/uploads/2017/12/BMS-Vision-02A. pdf
10. Women's Health Concern (2015) *The Menopause*. Marlow: WHC. www.womens-health-concern.org/help-and-advice/ factsheets/menopause
11. Freedman RR (2013) Menopausal hot flushes: mechanisms, endocrinology, treatment. *Journal of Steroid Biochemistry and Molecular Biology* 142: 115–20.
12. Cancer Research UK (2018) Hot flushes and sweats in women. www.cancerresearchuk.org/ about-cancer/coping/physically/sex-hormone-symptoms/women-coping-with-hormone-symptoms/hot-flushes-and-sweats.
13. Newson L (2019) Menopause survey results published! My Menopause Doctor, 12 March. www.menopausedoctor.co.uk/news/ menopause-survey-results-published
14. Scullin MK, Krueger ML, Ballard HK, et al. (2018) The effects of bedtime writing on difficulty falling asleep: a polysomnographic study comparing to-do lists and completed activity lists. *Journal of Experimental Psychology: General* 147(1): 139–46.
15. Migraine Trust (2019) Menopause and midlife. www.migrainetrust.org/about-migraine/trigger-factors/menopause-and-midlife.
16. Davis SR, Castelo-Branco C, Chedraui P, et al. (2012) Understanding weight gain at menopause. *Climacteric* 15(5): 419–29.
17. NHS Choices (2016) 'Why is my waist size important?' www.nhs.uk/common-health-questions/lifestyle/why-is-my-waist-size-important.
18. Saccomani S, Lui-Filho JF, Juliato CR, et al. (2017) Does obesity increase the risk of hot flushes among midlife women? A population-based study. *Menopause* 2017; 22(10): 1065–70.
19. NHS Choices (2016) Urinary incontinence: symptoms. www.nhs.uk/conditions/urinary-incontinence/symptoms.
20. NHS Choices (2018) Breast changes in older women. www.nhs.uk/live-well/healthy-body/ breast-changes-in-older-women.
21. American Academy of Dermatology (2019) Caring for your skin in menopause. www.aad. org/public/skin-hair-nails/skin-care/skin-care-during-menopause.
22. Rajpar S (2019) Menopause and hair loss (fact sheet). My Menopause Doctor. www. menopausedoctor.co.uk/menopause/ menopause-and-hair-loss-by-consultant-dermatologist-dr-sajjad-rajpar.
23. Peck T, Olsakovsky L, Aggarwal S (2017) Dry eye syndrome in menopause and perimenopausal age group. *Journal of Mid-Life Health* 8(2): 51–54.
24. Oral Health Foundation (2019) Burning mouth syndrome. www.dentalhealth.org/burning-mouth-syndrome.
25. Age UK (2019) Osteoporosis. www.ageuk.org. uk/information-advice/health-wellbeing/ conditions-illnesses/osteoporosis.
26. National Institute for Health and Care Excellence (2015) *Menopause: Diagnosis and Management*. NICE Guideline NG23. London: NICE. www.nice. org.uk/Guidance/NG23.
27. Hodis HN, Mack WJ, Henderson VW, et al. (2016) Vascular effects of early versus late postmenopausal treatment with estradiol. *New England Journal of Medicine* 374: 1221–31.
28. Maclaran K, Stevenson JC (2012) Primary

prevention of cardiovascular disease with HRT. *Women's Health (Lond)* 8: 63–74.

29. Women's Health Initiative (2019) Hormone therapy trials (HT). www.whi.org/about/SitePages/HT.aspx.

30. Breast Cancer Now (2016) Breast cancer facts. https://breastcancernow.org/about-breast-cancer/want-to-know-about-breast-cancer/breast-cancer-facts.

31a. NHS.uk (2018) Overview: HIV and AIDS. www.nhs.uk/conditions/hiv-and-aids

31b. Tariq S, Burns FM, Gilson R, et al (2019) PRIME (Positive Transitions Through the Menopause) Study: a protocol for a mixed-methods study investigating the impact of the menopause on the health and well-being of women living with HIV in England. BMJ Open 9:e025497. doi: 10.1136/bmjopen-2018-025497

32. Macmillan Cancer Support (2014) Cancer and the menopause. www.macmillan.org.uk/information-and-support/coping/side-effects-and-symptoms/menopause/cancer-and-menopause.html.

33. Coquoz A, Gruetter C, Stute P (2019) Impact of micronized progesterone on body weight, body mass index, and glucose metabolism: a systematic review. *Climacteric* 22: 148–61.

34. British Menopause Society (2019) *Bioidentical HRT*. BMS Consensus Statement. Marlow: BMS. https://thebms.org.uk/publications/consensus-statements/bioidentical-hrt.

35. British Menopause Society (2019) *Testosterone Replacement in Menopause*. Marlow: BMS. https://thebms.org.uk/publications/tools-for-clinicians/testosterone-replacement-in-menopause.

36. Baber RJ, Panay N, Fenton A, for the IMS Writing Group (2016) 2016 IMS Recommendations on women's midlife health and menopause hormone therapy, *Climacteric* 19: 109–50.

37. Mind (2017) Cognitive behavioural therapy. www.mind.org.uk/information-support/drugs-and-treatments/cognitive-behavioural-therapy-cbt/.

38. Driel, CM, Stuursma, A, Schroevers, MJ, et al. Mindfulness, cognitive behavioural and behaviour-based therapy for natural and treatment-induced menopausal symptoms: a systematic review and meta-analysis. *BJOG* 2019; 126: 330–39.

39. NHS (2018) Herbal medicines. www.nhs.uk/conditions/herbal-medicines.

40. Adrian W (2009) Western medical acupuncture: a definition. *Acupuncture in Medicine* 27(1): 33–35.

41. Royal College of Obstetricians and Gynaecologists (2018) *Treatment for Symptoms of the Menopause. Information for You.* London: RCOG. www.rcog.org.uk/en/patients/patient-leaflets/treatment-symptoms-menopause.

42. Weeks K (2017) Hillary Clinton used 'alternate nostril breathing' after her loss. Here's why you should, too. *Washington Post*, 15 September. www.washingtonpost.com/news/inspired-life/wp/2017/09/15/hillary-clinton-used-alternate-nostril-breathing-after-her-election-loss-heres-why-you-really-should-too.

43. Guthold R, Stevens GA, Riley LM, Bull FC (2018) Worldwide trends in insufficient physical activity from 2001 to 2016: a pooled analysis of 358 population-based surveys with 1.9 million participants. *Lancet Global Health* 6(10): PE1077–e1086.

44. Mishra N, Mishra VN, Devanshi (2011). Exercise beyond menopause: dos and don'ts. *Journal of Mid-Life Health* 2(2): 51–56.

45. Daley A, Stokes-Lampard H, Thomas A, MacArthur C (2014) Exercise for vasomotor menopausal symptoms. *Cochrane Database of Systematic Reviews* 2014(11): CD006108.

46. Blümel JE, Fica J, Chedraui P, et al. (2016) Sedentary lifestyle in middle-aged women is associated with severe menopausal symptoms and obesity. *Menopause* 23(5): 488–93.

47. NHS (2018) Physical activity guidelines for adults. www.nhs.uk/live-well/exercise.

48. Rackow P, Scholz U, Hornung R (2015) Received social support and exercising: an intervention study to test the enabling hypothesis. *British Journal of Health Psychology* 20: 763–76.

49. Public Health England (2016) *Government Dietary Recommendations: Government recommendations for energy and nutrients for males and females aged 1–18 years and 19+ years.* London: PHE. https://assets.publishing.service.gov.uk/government/system/uploads/attachment_data/file/618167/government_dietary_recommendations.pdf.

50. Cancer Research UK (2017) Vitamin D. www.cancerresearchuk.org/about-cancer/causes-of-cancer/sun-uv-and-cancer/vitamin-d.

51. Drinkaware (2019) UK alcohol unit guidance: CMO's low risk drinking guidelines. www.drinkaware.co.uk/alcohol-facts/alcoholic-drinks-units/latest-uk-alcohol-unit-guidance.

52. Public Health England, Food Standards Agency (2018) *National Diet and Nutrition Survey: results from years 7 and 8 (combined) of the rolling programme (2014/2015 to 2015/2016).* London: PHE. https://assets.publishing.service.gov.uk/government/uploads/system/uploads/attachment_data/file/699241/NDNS_results_years_7_and_8.pdf.

53. NHS (2017) Eat well. How does sugar in our diet affect our health? www.nhs.uk/live-well/eat-well/how-does-sugar-in-our-diet-affect-our-health.

54. NHS (2018) Probiotics. www.nhs.uk/conditions/probiotics.

55. British Menopause Society (2016) National survey: the results. https://thebms.org.uk/wp-content/uploads/2016/04/BMS-NationalSurvey-MARCH2017.pdf.

56. Irving G, Neves AL, Dambha-Miller H, et al. (2017) International variations in primary care physician consultation time: a systematic review of 67 countries. *BMJ Open* 7: e017902.

57. Greene J. (1976) A factor analytic study of climacteric symptoms. *Journal of Psychosomatic Research* 20: 425–30.

58. NICE (2015) Questions to ask about the menopause, in *Menopause Diagnosis and Management. Information for the Public.* London: NICE. www.nice.org.uk/guidance/ng23/ifp/chapter/Questions-to-ask-about-menopause.

59. Faculty of Sexual and Reproductive Healthcare (2017) *FSRH Guideline: Contraception for Women Aged Over 40 Years.* London: FSRH. www.fsrh.org/news/updated-clinical-guideline-published-contraception-for-women.

60. Office for National Statistics (2018) Divorces in England and Wales: 2017. www.ons.gov.uk/peoplepopulationandcommunity/birthsdeathsandmarriages/divorce/bulletins/divorcesinenglandandwales/2017#at-what-age-are-opposite-sex-couples-most-likely-to-divorce.

61. Cumming GP, Currie HD, Moncur R, Lee AJ (2009) Web-based survey on the effect of menopause on women's libido in a computer-literate population. *Menopause International* 15(1): 8–12.

62. Cabral, PU, Canário AC, Spyrides MH, et al. (2014) Physical activity and sexual function in middle-aged women. *Revista da Associação Médica Brasileira* 60(1): 47–52.

63. Hormone Health Network (2019) What is oxytocin? www.hormone.org/hormones-and-health/hormones/oxytocin.

64. Clark L, Stoneburner A, Bulkley J, et al. (2017) Genitourinary symptoms of menopause (GSM): impact on sexually active and inactive women (abstract S-6), 28th Annual Meeting of the North American Menopause Society October 11–14, 2017, Philadelphia, PA. Menopause 24(12): 1426.

65. Women's Health concern (2017) *Contraception for the Older Woman.* Marlow: WHC. www.womens-health-concern.org/help-and-advice/factsheets/contraception-older-woman.

66. FPA (2018) IUS (intrauterine system). https://sexwise.fpa.org.uk/contraception/ius-intrauterine-system.

67. British Society for Sexual Medicine (2017) A practical guide on the assessment and management of testosterone deficiency in adult men. www.bssm.org.uk/wp-content/uploads/2018/02/BSSM-Practical-Guide-High-Res-single-pp-view-final.pdf.

68. Office for National Statistics (2019) Birth characteristics in England and Wales: 2017. www.ons.gov.uk/peoplepopulationandcommunity/birthsdeathsandmarriages/livebirths/bulletins/birthcharacteristicsinenglandandwales/2017.

69. NHS (2018) Exercise: Physical activity guidelines for children and young people. www.nhs.uk/live-well/exercise/physical-activity-guidelines-children-and-young-people.

70. Government Equalities Office (2017) Menopause transition: effects on women's economic participation. www.gov.uk/government/publications/menopause-transition-effects-on-womens-economic-participation.

71. Scottish National Party (2019) Together we are working together to break down barriers and advance equality for all. www.snp.org/together-we-are-working-to-break-down-barriers-and-advance-equality-for-all.

72. Nuffield Health (2014) One in four with menopause symptoms concerned about ability to cope with life. www.nuffieldhealth.com/article/one-in-four-with-menopause-symptoms-concerned-about-ability-to-cope-with-life.

73. Griffiths A, Maclennan S, Wong YYV (2010) Women's Experience of Working through the Menopause. Nottingham: British Occupational Health Research Foundation. www.bohrf.org.uk/downloads/Womens_Experience_of_Working_through_the_Menopause-Dec_2010.pdf.

74. Faculty of Occupational Medicine of the Royal College of Physicians (2016) *Guidance on Menopause and the Workplace.* London: FOM. www.fom.ac.uk/wp-content/uploads/Guidance-on-menopause-and-the-workplace-v6.pdf.

75. Trades Union Congress (2013) *Supporting Working Women through the Menopause: Guidance for Union Representatives.* London: TUC. www.tuc.org.uk/sites/default/files/TUC_menopause_0.pdf.

76. Sianoja M, Syrek CJ, de Bloom J, Ket al. (2018) Enhancing daily well-being at work through lunchtime park walks and relaxation exercises: recovery experiences as mediators. *Journal of Occupational Health Psychology* 23(3): 428–42.

77. Health and Safety Executive (2019) Should VDU users be given breaks? www.hse.gov.uk/contact/faqs/vdubreaks.htm.

78. Wales Trades Union Congress (2019) Adjustment passport. www.tuc.org.uk/exampledisabilityadjustmentpassport.

79. Women's Health Concern (2017) *HRT.* Marlow: WHS. www.womens-health-concern.org/help-and-advice/factsheets/hrt.

80. Women's Health Concern (2017) *Vaginal Dryness.* Marlow: WHS. www.womens-health-concern.org/help-and-advice/factsheets/vaginal-dryness.

Index

Acknowledgements

This book has been a huge amount of work which I have not been able to do alone. I would like to thank Kat Keogh, who is the contributing editor for this work. She has worked tirelessly with me to ensure the content is accurate, evidence based and up to date.

I work with an incredible team of people in my clinic who constantly and patiently listen to my relentless ideas to improve menopause care for women which is so desperately needed. My clinical partner, Rebecca Lewis, is a pillar of strength to me and my business mentor Marcus Daly continues to teach and educate me. Paul Isaacs has given me the confidence to continue with my venture. Kate, Abigail and Linda are amazing friends and continue to give me encouragement and enthusiasm towards my work.

My husband Paul never fails to believe in my passion to help women and supports me both at home and at work. He is my rock and provides me strength and confidence to believe in myself. I would also like to acknowledge my family, especially Jessica, Sophie, Lucy, Annie, Sarah, John and Kay, who constantly encourage me in so many ways to continue with my mission of educating as many people as possible about the menopause.

Finally I would like to thank all my patients and the many women who follow me on social media who have told me so many stories about their menopause experience – they have all helped give me support and energy to produce this book!

Louise Newson, September 2019